SEARCHING FOR A CURE

SEARCHING FOR A CURE

National Health Policy Considered

Jonas Morris

PICA PRESS
New York

The author thanks Simon and Schuster for permission to use quotations from *Governing America: An Insider's Report from the White House and the Cabinet,* by Joseph A. Califano, Jr., copyright 1981 by Joseph A. Califano, Jr.

Published in the United States of America in 1984 by
PICA PRESS
Distributed by Universe Books
381 Park Avenue South, New York, N.Y. 10016

84 85 86 87 88 / 10 9 8 7 6 5 4 3 2 1

Printed in the United States of America

Library of Congress No. 83-040568
ISBN 0-87663-741-1

For my parents
Charles and Dorothy Morris

CONTENTS

PREFACE

This book is designed for the general reader, one who is concerned about how our federal government makes domestic policy. But it also is designed for those who, because of their work or interests, are concerned specifically about the making of national health policy and for students training for professions in or related to the health care field. The book examines the impact of federal policy upon the health care system, and why that policy is what it is.

The focus of the book is on efforts over the past twenty years to begin a program of national health insurance (NHI), and on how and why those efforts have come to naught. But because the campaign for NHI is only the most visible aspect of national health policy, the book attempts to reach beyond to explore other major aspects of the making of that policy. The history of the federal involvement in delivering and supporting health care and related efforts is described as a way of giving a more detailed view of how federal policy has developed.

The book also examines the impact that technological developments in the health care arena are having on national health policy and the problems that are on the horizon if the federal government continues to absorb the cost of very expensive care for a relatively small group of people, such as it does for those with kidney disease. It is a very touchy issue.

The book defines federal health policy narrowly: providing or supporting health care, the training of health care personnel, and support for biomedical research, and other related efforts such as planning for health services. This is essentially the way the federal budget defines health. But even within this definition federal health policy is an enormous subject and one book cannot conceivably cover all its facets; this one is no exception.

I am a journalist by trade, although I have not always earned my living this way. For more than a decade I published a newsletter—*Health Systems Report*—on federal health policy, and this book is an outgrowth of that experience. For about eight years, ending in 1977, I was also, in addition to publishing and writing about federal health policy, a lobbyist representing the independent, nonprofit community mental health centers. Thus, the portions of this book on the mental health centers program are not written from a purely unbiased point of view, although I hope, and believe, distance has made the heart grow less fond.

INTRODUCTION

The health care industry is one of the biggest in this country in terms of total expenditures and personnel employed, and through it the American people and their government currently spend about $325 billion each year.

But the health care industry has a financial structure like no other major American industry. The triangle of patient, physician and insurance company paying for care, which usually insulates the patient from much of the cost of health care, largely nullifies the traditional competitive forces of the marketplace that are the hallmark of United States business.

The patient does not in most cases purchase care from a hospital but instead purchases access to hospitals by buying health insurance. In a similar manner, insurance provides access to physicians for treatment of major illnesses or disabilities. Some insurance may cover the cost of virtually all health care. Thus, the patient—the consumer—makes little effort to have the provider keep prices down. He wants only all the care necessary to make him well, as long as his insurance will pay the cost.

It is, in large part, this phenomenon that has caused health costs to rise so dramatically in recent years. Although the federal government pays a large share of the nation's health care bill—nearly 50 percent—in one way or another, it has been nearly powerless to check this rise.

Clearly, one of the responsibilities of government can be assuring access to health care for its people. To what extent the United States government should assume that responsibility has been a major topic of debate over the past two decades. It is not a debate that will soon be concluded.

The nation has the capacity, in terms of resources, knowledge and ability, to assure every citizen access to the highest-quality health care ever known to mankind. That we have chosen not to do so is not necessarily a reflection of our lack of caring for our fellow countrymen, but rather, in part, a manifestation of our pluralistic political system and our way of developing social policy.

In part, also, though, it is a reflection of the difficulties involved in doing so—the cost, the administrative problems, and, perhaps more than any other reason, a quandary over where, once the commitment is fully made, the obligation to preserve life would stop. The latter has not so much to do with providing vaccinations, financing the construction of and equipping hospitals, or paying for routine operations, although that is part of it, as it does with moving forward the frontiers of our life-saving abilities, most notably artificial organs, organ transplants or procedures such as dialysis for the person whose kidneys have failed. These procedures often are very expensive for both the public purse and the individual person and may extend life only a few years.

Thus, a major element in the nation's health policy debate, although rarely, if ever, so articulated, is how far we want to reach toward immortality.

The one clear reality for man since the beginning of human life has been the knowledge that one day he would die. But the one clear desire of almost all humans has been to live as long as possible. Forever for many is not too long, and the exotic medical procedures of today, such as the artificial heart or the transplanted natural heart, make immortality much more possible, in one's fantasy, than it ever has been. Who can predict how the fantasy will be encouraged by the medical procedure of tomorrow?

This dilemma—to what extent the federal government should promise all citizens the longest life possible—is at the core, though seldom recognized as such, of our nation's debate over the size and shape of federal health policy. In large part, the public's perception of what it should get from the federal government in the way of health care has been pushed forward by those political leaders who have argued that the best in health care is a right of citizenship and thus ensuring it a responsibility of a government such as ours. In part, the promise of freedom from worry over health care costs has been a staple in the rhetoric of some national leaders, and clearly it has been an attractive morsel to offer the voters. Since the federal government does not go broke, there has seemed little risk involved in pushing it into this commitment.

The symbol of high expectations in health services has been national health insurance, a term much bantered about for nearly fifty years and one that can be defined in many different ways. Loosely, however, it has come to mean a federally sponsored program that ensures every citizen access to the health care he or she may need. NHI is a prospect, regardless of how it is defined, that today is still far from materializing. A decade ago it seemed that a program of some sort of national health insurance was only a matter of time; now there seems the strong likelihood that one may never come into being.

Many barriers have stood in the way of creating a national health insurance program. The biggest has been the substantial rise in the cost of health care, and particularly of hospital care, over the past decade and a half. Elected officials have agreed that this rise, coupled with an economy under severe stress, make the enactment of a program of national health insurance unacceptable at the moment, for it would be too costly.

Yet, it is legitimate to ask how much for health care is too much. As a nation, we spend nearly as much on jewelry and clothing each year as we do on health care, but the nation's expenditure for these commodities is not the subject of national debate as is that for health care. It is only because health care has become heavily financed by public dollars that it has taken on this controversial role.

PROLOGUE

In the early spring of 1980 Jimmy Carter and Ted Kennedy were in combat for the Democratic Party's presidential nomination for that fall's election.

Each by then had put forward the details of his national health insurance program, and it looked as if Congress might actually get serious about NHI, for Russell Long, then chairman of the Senate Finance Committee, had rekindled his interest in the subject and put forth a plan of his own. Long's interest, because of his control of the Finance Committee through which the legislation must pass, was needed to put national health insurance high enough on the political agenda to win enactment, and now that prospect seemed nearly a reality.

But Long's interest would not be enough. The two major combatants would not be able to see their way to compromising their differences over national health insurance, although their differences were by then small in comparison to what they once had been.

So the spring and summer of 1980 and the fall, too, passed without Congress enacting a national health insurance program, and Jimmy Carter left the White House in defeat to his successor, Ronald Reagan.

With that change, the federal government's attitude toward national health insurance changed radically. The White House was now unalterably opposed. Whether NHI might again rebound easily to a top spot on the presidential and congressional agenda once Reagan left office would be determined by the topsy-turvy character of American politics.

The story of how the nation's government considered a health program that might have ensured everyone access to adequate health care must be told within the context of the entire federal apparatus for making federal health policy. It must also be told within the context of the American political system, and particularly of the four-year cycle of presidential campaigns that leaves each president no more than eighteen months in which to push successfully for enactment of major new programs before political forces are largely neutralized in anticipation of first the midterm congressional elections and then the next presidential election.

The larger universe for making health policy includes the rest of the government's responsibilities for health: Medicare and Medicaid, the veterans and military health care programs, the federal government's health insurance program for its own employees, federal support for biomedical research, the investment the federal government makes in the nation's health care system through tax laws, and—during an earlier era—a wide variety of categorical programs that targeted federal funds on specific health needs.

The story also needs to be told within the context of the high inflation of health care costs over the past fifteen years, the federal government's efforts to influence the way the health care industry works, and the ever-growing size of the health care industry that by 1983 had reached $325 billion.

But if national health insurance is only one part of the story of the federal government and health, it is, nevertheless, the political barometer of the health field. As the political climate changes so that, for whatever reasons, NHI becomes more feasible, congressional health leaders and others in Congress start introducing their own national health insurance proposals, as much to protect their own interests as for any other reason. As the idea becomes less attractive because of fiscal, ideological or other reasons, ardor for NHI wanes.

National health insurance by the mid-1970s had become the litmus test by which Democratic presidential candidates had their commitment to liberal dogma measured. In 1974, NHI appeared to be an attainable legislative accomplishment, and thus by 1976 Democrats running for president would have to show their allegiance to a strong federal national health insurance program in order to win liberal, and particularly labor, backing. This was the reality Jimmy Carter faced in 1975 as he moved forward with his own presidential campaign, and he finally made such a commitment that won him the support of labor in several critical primaries, such as Florida, Michigan and Pennsylvania. It would be a commitment on which labor, and Ted Kennedy, would later say he welshed. National health insurance had become a pawn to be used in the chess game of political ambitions, and all else the federal government did with regard to the development of health policy was being drawn into that whirlpool.

1
THE EARLY YEARS

Efforts to develop a program of national health insurance are generally regarded to have been first initiated during the 1930s as part of proposals for a system of social security. In reality, the seeds for comprehensive care guaranteed by the federal government go back to the founding days of the Republic.

Early in the first administration of George Washington, the federal government took action to deal with the threat of epidemics. By 1798 Congress presented President John Adams with legislation establishing federal responsibility for the health of merchant seamen, who were bringing contagious diseases to America's shores and causing epidemics. That program, which became the foundation of today's Public Health Service, the principal federal agency involved in health issues, established a medical care system for an entire class of citizens and financed that care with payments withheld from wages.

The first identifiable effort by a president, however, to extend the federal responsibility for health care to all Americans appear to have been made by Woodrow Wilson. On March 4, 1913, Wilson in his first inaugural address called for defining the federal government's responsibility for ensuring health care for all citizens.

He said the nation had not "studied and perfected the means by which government may be put at the service of humanity, in safeguarding the health of the nation, the health of its men and its women and its children, as well as their rights in the struggle for existence. This is no sentimental duty. The firm basis of government is justice, not pity. These are matters of justice."[1] The extent of his concern, while there, was obscure, and he might not even have gone this far if one of his opponents, Theodore Roosevelt, in the previous fall's campaign had not advocated national health insurance.

The view that the federal government should assume a role in providing health care for everyone sprang from the liberal ideology that grew out of concerns for the welfare of the poor, the jobless, the disabled and others who were having difficulty caring fully for themselves.

The strength of the Progressive movement and support for a national health care program, however, faded, and for a number of reasons. World War I deflected attention of the country from social concerns. Also, the American Medical Association, which had initially backed plans for government-sponsored health insurance, toward the end of the decade changed its position after a change in leadership and by 1920 opposed the idea. This new stance would become the organization's permanent posture; from now on the AMA would strongly oppose most significant new federal ventures in the health arena on the grounds that they would jeopardize the delicate relationship between doctor and patient and lead to socialized medicine. But another force for opposition developed as well. Some elements within the labor movement began opposing government-sponsored health insurance fearing that it would weaken the movement. Workers covered by a government health insurance program would not be as dependent upon labor unions in their struggle with employers.[2]

The New Deal Years

It was not until the emergence of the New Deal in 1933 that proposals for national health insurance again surfaced. President Franklin Roosevelt was sympathetic to the idea, and early in his administration there seemed to be the strong possibility that the proposal would be woven into what became his recommendations for a social security retirement program. But national health insurance was not near the top of his agenda for social change. Although he spoke favorably of the concept on a number of occasions, he would not actually put forward a plan before he died in April 1945.

An early version of what later became the administration's proposal for social security contained a provision establishing a social insurance board responsible for making recommendations on, among other issues, health insurance. But that charge was subsequently removed, and when Roosevelt in 1935 sent his social security message to Congress he said he was "not at this time recommending the adoption of so-called health insurance, although groups representing the medical profession are cooperating with the federal government in the further study of the subject, and definite progress is being made."[3]

There were several reasons why Roosevelt did not then recommend national health insurance. The first was political: a fear that the baggage of NHI would encumber the social security retirement program and jeopardize its passage. Another was substantive: a concern that the existing health care system was not capable of taking on the task of NHI and that this system first needed to be strengthened through other types of federal support before national health insurance was enacted. This latter concern was one that would surface again and again over the years as NHI was considered in both the Executive Branch and Congress.

Furthermore, Roosevelt was also pushing for enactment of an unemployment compensation program, and Frances Perkins, his secretary of labor, along with organized labor opposed any proposals, such as national health insurance, that would compete with that plan.

But, when the social security act was signed into law on August 14, 1935, even though it did not create a national health insurance program, it did authorize funds for federal grants to states, to be matched by an equal amount in state funds, for developing local public health and disease prevention programs and for providing health care to mothers and children. Although this was not the first authority for federal support for health service programs, the commitment was now solid, and from this point on until the 1980s the federal government's role in providing and paying for health care would only grow.

However, in the Roosevelt years, the idea of national health insurance continued to receive some attention. In 1939, Robert Wagner, a Democratic senator from New York, sponsored a national health bill that carried the final proposal of an interdepartmental committee established to consider further changes to the social security act. The Wagner bill would have provided a more substantial program of health care for infants and mothers and expanded other federal support to states for health care services. But it was a proposal that found little support elsewhere in Congress.

Early in the next decade the initiative shifted to Congress and repeatedly during the 1940s legislation was introduced to establish a national health insurance program in one form or another. Congressional sponsors of national health insurance during the 1940s were all Democrats, for then as today their attitude toward NHI was a quick way of distinguishing broadly between the two major political parties. Wagner and his colleague James Murray of Montana sponsored legislation in the Senate, while John Dingell of Michigan proposed the measure in the House. Their bill created a program that mandated health insurance for everyone in the country. It would be paid for by a payroll tax similar to that which financed the social security retirement system. The Murray-Wagner-Dingell bill, even though it was exclusively a financing scheme, became the prototype for latter-day national health insurance legislation.

In November 1945, eight months into his presidency, Harry Truman called on Congress to enact a national health insurance program similar to that proposed by Wagner, Murray and Dingell, and the NHI initiative shifted to the White House. The new president repeated his calls for NHI almost on a yearly basis. In 1949, following his election victory and the resumption of control of Congress by the Democrats, Truman came out strongly for national health insurance in his State of the Union message and later that spring sent a special message to Congress reoffering the plan he had put forward earlier. Unlike previous years there was serious congressional consideration in 1949 and hearings produced some bitter controversy between proponents and opponents. By this time, too, proponents, spearheaded by organized labor, had banded together to form the Committee for the Nation's Health, which included such prominent individuals as Eleanor Roosevelt. But by the end of Truman's presidency there had been no meaningful action on the request, and national health insurance as such was to lie dormant until Medicare was enacted in 1965.

If no agreement could be reached on the need for health insurance for everyone, in the years following World War II a consensus did begin to emerge within both political parties that the federal government had a responsibility to ensure that the health care needs of the poor were taken care of. The distinction between federally financed health care for the poor as opposed to care for everyone, however, was not simply one of degree; it was fundamental, for it went to how this aid should be financed.

Those who supported a comprehensive national health insurance program covering everyone—and this was the Wagner-Murray-Dingell bill—wanted the aid financed through a payroll tax. As such it would become an entitlement for which the beneficiary would have already paid and thus one that could not be taken away, at least not easily. Those who wanted to limit federal aid for health care to the poor would finance that aid out of the general revenues of the Treasury and distribute it through grants to the states. This type of aid would be subject to the vagaries of annual appropriations by Congress.

Under the first approach, that of liberal Democrats, a person would have a vested right that gave him inalienable access to the main stream of health care. Under the other approach, that of conservatives and most Republicans, the person would receive a charity donation that put him in a separate class from others where he could get a special, but perhaps less desirable, level of care.

This distinction began to be articulated soon after Truman started pushing aggressively for enactment of an NHI program. In 1946, Robert Taft, from Ohio, perhaps the most esteemed Republican in the Senate at that time, sponsored legislation providing grants to states so that they could pay for medical care for the poor, and in fact this proposal was endorsed by the American Medical Association, which was then and has remained the principal opponent of comprehensive national health insurance. But as Taft introduced his health care plan for the poor, he argued that Truman's proposal not only would result in "the socialization of medicine, but it is a complete nationalization of the medical profession."[4] Truman countered by maintaining that the socialism tag did not apply since doctors would not become federal employees and everyone would still be free to choose their own doctors. Taft's characterization, to be used later by others, was to be a convenient ploy, and through the years it has contributed to the success of those who have opposed a Truman-like plan.

In 1950, Taft's proposal finally found its way into law when the Social Security Act was amended to provide aid to states to help them pay for some of the cost of medical care to some of the poor, those who were beneficiaries of one of the various welfare programs. Federal aid to the poor prior to 1950, which took the form of grants to states that were then turned into cash assistance, went only for living expenses. The new approach was intended to provide health care at an earlier stage to a group of persons who often required more costly health care than others because they would not usually get care until the illness or disability had become serious.

President Truman, the first president to actually propose a national health insurance program, in December 1951 as he was starting his last year in office created a Commission on the Health Needs of the Nation. A year later, after his successor had been chosen, the commission filed its report, *Building America's Health,* and advocated a joint federal-state system for financing health care—a modest recommendation considering Truman's more sweeping proposal. But the panel also set the stage for greater federal involvement in health care in other ways.

It urged that federal funds be made available to medical schools and other health care training facilities to enable them to expand their facilities and to provide financial aid to medical students. It also urged more federal aid for the construction and improvement of hospitals, development of prepaid health plans, more federal support for the prevention of disease, and expanded support—both public and private—for biomedical research.[5]

With the election of Dwight Eisenhower in 1952, however, the chance, for the time being, of enacting of a national health insurance program, or even for significant expansion of existing programs, was gone, for the new president opposed NHI on very specific philosophical grounds. To Eisenhower, as for Taft, it was socialized medicine.

By 1953, when supporters of a comprehensive national health insurance program had given up hope for enactment of such a program, they narrowed their focus—they wanted instead an expansion of the social security program to provide health insurance, but only for the cost of hospital care, for the elderly, the same group that was covered by the retirement program. This was a group that was particularly needy. The elderly had higher than usual health care costs, particularly for long-term care and for chronic illnesses, yet their incomes were lower than most, and they were unable to purchase health insurance because of their higher liability and because they did not have easy access to group plans through employers. Legislation to establish such a program was introduced in 1953 and in subsequent years by Murray in the Senate and in the House again by Dingell along with his colleague Emanuel Celler, a Democrat from New York City. By 1957, however, the leadership for this effort had shifted to Amie Forand, a Democratic representative from Rhode Island, who sat on the Ways and Means Committee, the House committee that had responsibility for such legislation.

Although the Forand proposal became the marching rod for those who earlier had pushed Truman's plan and the lightning rod for those who opposed it, there was no serious action on it until 1960, when it became an issue in the presidential campaign. The Eisenhower administration countered with its own plan to help the elderly poor meet some of their health care costs, a plan that it dubbed Medicare. Under this plan, the federal government would make grants to the states, which would be matched by those states, to help them pay for certain specified health care costs, including hospital and nursing home costs, for the aged who were on welfare. It went further toward securing needed health care for the elderly poor than the 1950 legislation that applied to the poor regardless of age.

In March of 1960, the House Ways and Means Committee voted down the Forand bill by a substantial two-to-one margin. The panel's chairman, Wilbur Mills, a generally conservative Democrat from Arkansas, voted against it. Instead, the committee adopted a measure, designed by Mills, similar to Eisenhower's proposal, but with a significant difference—it included as beneficiaries elderly persons who did not qualify for welfare but needed help with their medical bills or they would likely become welfare beneficiaries. The Mills proposal was attached to an omnibus social security package the committee was considering, and that measure was passed by the full House in June 1960. This strategy was a way of undercutting the momentum. It was a typical tactic employed through the years: Enact a modest program to take the heat off for a larger one.

When Congress reconvened in the late summer of 1960 after the recess for the political conventions, the scene shifted to the Senate where the Democratic nominee, John Kennedy, said passage of the Forand bill was one of the top items on his political agenda for the tail-end session. The Forand bill, however, was turned down by the Finance Committee, which instead beefed up the provisions in the House bill. The legislation finally enacted was called the Kerr-Mills bill, for Mills and Robert Kerr, a Democratic senator from Oklahoma and the ranking Democrat, next to the chairman, on the Finance Committee.

Now federal aid for health care would go not only to the poor, through the 1950 program of state grants, but, in the case of the elderly, to the near-poor as well.

The election of John Kennedy, a liberal Democrat, to the presidency did not change significantly the composition of Congress, which during the postwar years had been dominated by a conservative coalition of Republicans and southern Democrats, and the new president's liberal proposals would have to seek compromise with this force.

Once in the White House, however, Kennedy again pushed for enactment of the Forand bill, now the King-Anderson bill for its new sponsors, Cecil King of California in the House and Clinton Anderson of New Mexico in the Senate. This measure, like the Forand bill before it, covered only hospital costs—not outpatient or physician services—for all the elderly regardless of their economic well-being. The measure made no significant progress in either 1961 or 1962. In June 1962, however, it was considered on the Senate floor when Anderson proposed it as an amendment to a pending welfare bill. The measure was defeated by a 52–48 roll call vote when Republicans and southern Democrats joined together in opposition. The closeness of the vote, however, was an indication that the proposal's time was coming.

President Kennedy put the measure forward again in 1963 after a new Congress convened, but there was no action on it before he was murdered in late November. It was not until 1964 with Lyndon Johnson in the White House that Congress began to look seriously at the proposal. The measure was ignored when the House that year wrote a social security bill, and then it was turned down by the Finance Committee. But it was adopted by a 49–44 roll call vote by the full Senate. When House and Senate conferees met to attempt to reconcile the differences, the two sides found themselves deadlocked, and the whole measure went under when Congress adjourned in the fall for the presidential elections. The stage was now fully set for enactment of today's Medicare program.

A clear possibility for Johnson after he won so handsomely in 1964 was to jump past Medicare and push for enactment of a full-fledged national health insurance program, as had been originally proposed by Wagner, Murray and Dingell. But that did not seem to be politically possible at the time, even with Johnson's considerable electoral strength behind him. Health was only one item on Johnson's political agenda. By 1965 the Vietnam war was starting to consume more and more of his attention, and the budgetary as well as political decisions involved were staring him in the face.

Furthermore, it might not be so easy to win enactment of a national health insurance program even if everything was going right. Organized medicine, in the form of the American Medical Association, had proven itself a formidable lobby in preventing the enactment of Medicare, and in the House Johnson still had a somewhat reluctant Ways and Means chairman, Wilbur Mills, to deal with. It was best, everyone thought then, to win enactment of Medicare, for which there was already considerable momentum, and then go on to push for passage of a comprehensive national health insurance program. It was, once again, the incremental approach.

If the election to the presidency first of John Kennedy and then of Lyndon Johnson set the stage for enactment of Medicare, it also opened up opportunity for creation of many of other federal health programs. In their combination these programs paved the way for a national health insurance program by building a stronger base of health care services (a need earlier articulated by Franklin Roosevelt) and by lessening the need for NHI in the sense that more people, young and old, poor and well-off, were getting most, if not all, of the health care they needed. This accomplishment frustrated liberal Democrats, for these programs were ones they strongly advocated, yet at the same time they saw them as complicating the drive for a larger national system of health care, one that, regardless of what it was called, would provide full health services for everyone.

Who's in Charge? Congress and the Executive Branch

Responsibility for health is spread far and wide throughout the federal establishment. In the Executive Branch, two departments (Health and Human Services, and Defense) and one agency (Veterans Administration) are responsible for multibillion-dollar health programs and many other departments and agencies have health responsibilities. In Congress, six committees have major responsibilities for health issues, and at least a half-dozen more also have responsibilities in the health area. This spread of responsibility throughout the two branches of government has been, in part, responsible for creating a tug-of-war between Congress and the administration over which shall have the dominant say in the development of health policy.

Although health issues in the Executive Branch are parceled out among numerous departments and agencies, the one with the most responsibility is the Department of Health and Human Services, or, until 1980, the Department of Health, Education and Welfare.

Until the 1960s, the department's responsibilities were easily organized into several discrete areas. The Public Health Service was then the lead agency on health matters, and its primary responsibilities were fostering state preventive health programs and running the federal government's biomedical research effort. Control over the development and marketing of new drugs was vested in the Food and Drug Administration (FDA), which originally was part of the Department of Agriculture. In 1940, the FDA was shifted to the Federal Security Administration, the predecessor of the Department of Health, Education and Welfare, where it was made a part of the Public Health Service.

The biomedical research program, begun in the early days of the Public Health Service, really got its start in 1937 when the first cancer act was passed establishing the National Cancer Institute. Since then, the National Institutes of Health has grown to become the preeminent biomedical research establishment in the world, and by 1983 the federal government was investing $4 billion annually in the effort.

The National Institutes of Health became and has continued to be an extremely important element in federal health policy because it is responsible not only for increasing understanding of the human body through biomedical research but also for translating improved understanding into better care. While other health programs have absorbed a larger share of the health care budget, the biomedical research program has remained the primary vehicle for finding solutions to health care dilemmas.

Outside the Department of Health and Human Services, the Department of Defense and the Veterans Administration had their own health programs to provide care to their particular constituencies. There was a smattering of other health programs throughout the federal establishment, most with the focus of providing care but some with other foci, such as protecting the public from harmful radiation or bad meat. But by and large, until the 1960s, matters of health were not the responsibility of the federal government; rather they were the responsibility of state and local governments or the private sector.

In the early 1960s, the federal government's relationship to health, particularly the responsibility of providing or financing health care, began to change, and by the end of that decade the difference was so vast that comparison was difficult.

The changes of the mid-1960s also had other ramifications. They substantially altered the way health issues were perceived within the Executive Branch. The emergence of the federal government as a principal in financing health care through Medicare (the federal program of health care for the elderly) and Medicaid (the federal-state program of health care for the poor) caused all other health responsibilities of the federal government to take on new dimensions. Furthermore, the new dimensions caused the emergence of a set of conflicting vectors representing different federal health responsibilities.

By the end of the 1960s, the federal government had become a major purchaser of health care as, in effect, an insurance company for Medicare and Medicaid beneficiaries. By then it was also a major purchaser of health insurance through its federal employees health benefits program. In addition, the federal government was the largest provider of health care in the country because of the services it delivered directly to veterans, current and retired military personnel and their dependents, federal prisoners, merchant seamen and other select groups. Finally, through a number of specialized grant programs (several dozen of which were enacted in the 1960s and 1970s), the federal government helped finance care delivered by state and local governments and private agencies. In addition to its role in the delivery of care and biomedical research, the federal government was heavily involved in training health care personnel, constructing hospitals, planning for the use of health care resources, and regulating research and development of drugs, health care equipment and supplies. All of this, even by 1970, gave the federal government major leverage over the health care industry. Today, that leverage is even more substantial.

The division of responsibilities for health issues within Congress emerged over the years largely because of the way Congress is structured—a collection of individual fiefdoms, each member virtually autonomous, responsible, in most regards, only to the constituents who elect him.

Congressional committees, the places where health programs are created, revised or given funds with which to operate, are, in one sense, mini-congresses. Each has its own rules, although patterned after the rules of the chamber of which it is a product. Each assigns members to its subcommittees and elects its own leaders and the leaders of its subcommittees. Members get assigned to a committee by the caucus of their chamber's party, although seniority plays a large role.

Control of legislative responsibility is the key to power in Congress, and legislative responsibility, at least in the initial stages of development, is almost entirely exercised through committees and subcommittees.

While virtually any committee of Congress can find an excuse to work on health issues if it wants to—the Aging committees because of Medicare, the Veterans and Armed Services committees because of the military and veterans health programs, Governmental Operations because of general oversight—there are six that have a predominant influence, and they tend to compete with one another. Over major health legislation, such as national health insurance, there is often dual responsibility.

In the House, the Energy and Commerce Committee has jurisdiction over the Public Health Service, Medicaid, and part of Medicare. The Ways and Means Committee, because of its responsibility for tax matters, has charge of that part of Medicare that is financed by a payroll tax, and shares the rest with the Commerce Committee. They both have jurisdiction over national health insurance. Both have health subcommittees where the initial work generally, but not always, goes on. The third House committee is Appropriations, which has charge of writing the annual appropriations act for all government agencies, and its subcommittee on labor, health, education and welfare does the initial work on the health budget.

When writing legislation creating new or expanding existing Public Health Service programs, such as federal support for training physicians, running community health clinics or carrying out biomedical research, the Commerce Committee establishes the goals for the programs, sets the guidelines for its operation and puts limits called authorizations on the amount of money that might be appropriated for it. It also from time to time reviews the operations of the programs—called oversight—to see whether they are being run the way it had intended. The Ways and Means Committee operates much the same way, although the amount of money spent each year for the one health program over which it has jurisdiction—Medicare—is determined by the number of beneficiaries who needed care and how much care they needed; thus the usual appropriations process does not apply. The Appropriations Committee has its say in determining health policy by proposing a specific budget each year for those health programs, like biomedical research, that do not get automatic appropriations.

In the Senate, the makeup is similar to that in the House, where three committees dominate: The Labor and Human Resources Committee is analogous in jurisdiction to the House Commerce panel except that it does not have any responsibility for Medicare or Medicaid (Finance does). The Finance Committee parallels the Ways and Means Committee because of its responsibility for tax issues. The Appropriations Committee has identical responsibilities to its companion panel in the House.

And then there are the Budget committees that propose in their annual budget resolutions the targets for health spending for the upcoming fiscal year—targets under which each of the six major committees work.

Power in Congress is largely in direct proportion to a member's committee membership and responsibility thereon. Since health is such a wide-ranging field and has such a substantial impact on the federal budget, chairmanship of health subcommittees is often a strongly sought-after post, but not always.

Although committees and their subcommittees operate on the democratic principle—one member, one vote—the chairman can be very influential if he wants to be. His formal powers include those of convening and adjourning the panel and setting the agenda; beyond these he can develop coalitions and sense when the time is ripe to push a bill forward. The House since 1953 has been controlled by Democrats, and thus all committee and subcommittee chairmen have been Democrats.

The chairmanship of the Commerce health subcommittee from 1971 until 1978 when he retired from Congress was held by Paul Rogers, who represented Palm Beach, Florida. Actually, Rogers had been running the subcommittee for four years prior to the time he assumed the chairmanship, when John Jarman from Tulsa, Oklahoma, had the title. But Jarman was a lazy man and let Rogers run the show; it was good experience for Rogers because he had control of the panel during the Johnson era when so many health programs were enacted.

When Rogers retired from Congress in 1978 he was succeeded by Henry Waxman, a liberal from Los Angeles who campaigned aggressively to win the spot and jump over in seniority several colleagues on the subcommittee. In fact, Waxman was working so hard to win the chairmanship that he neglected to pay sufficient attention to who was being assigned to the subcommittee in 1979, and he ended up with a very conservative panel that was difficult for him to control at times.

While the health subcommittee of Commerce was very attractive, that was not to be the case in Ways and Means, where members found it more frustrating than desirable. There had been no subcommittees on Ways and Means during Wilbur Mills's tenure as chairman, but when Al Ullman, an Oregonian, took over in 1975 he created them, and the health panel that year went to Dan Rostenkowski, from Chicago, who was to succeed Ullman as chairman of the full committee in 1981. Rostenkowski in 1977 was to have the task of shepherding through

Carter's hospital cost containment bill, a task that he obviously did not enjoy, and so when the chairmanship of another subcommittee opened up in 1979 Rostenkowski grabbed it, leaving the health subcommittee to Charles Rangel, a Harlem Democrat. Two years chairing the subcommittee was enough for Rangel, and in 1981 he, too, gave up the job, this time to Andrew Jacobs of Indiana.

In the Senate, Herman Talmadge of Georgia chaired the Finance health subcommittee from the time of its creation in 1973 until he was defeated for reelection in 1980. But often health legislation in Finance was written in the full committee where, until 1981, the chairman was Russell Long.

The other Senate panel with responsibility for writing health laws, the health subcommittee of the Labor and Human Services Committee (which earlier had been called the Labor and Public Welfare Committee), was chaired from 1971 until 1981, when the Democrats lost control, by Edward Kennedy, and of course served as the base for his efforts on national health insurance. For the two years prior to Kennedy's taking over, the subcommittee was chaired by Ralph Yarborough of Texas, and before that, for more than a decade, by Lister Hill of Alabama. Hill during this period also chaired the Senate Appropriations subcommittee that wrote the annual funding bill for the Department of Health, Education and Welfare, giving him substantial leverage over the fate of health programs. In 1981, the new chairman of the full committee, Orrin Hatch, a GOP senator from Utah, disbanded the health subcommittee.

The Appropriations subcommittee in the House for many years was chaired by the flamboyant Daniel Flood from Wilkes-Barre, Pennsylvania. He had succeeded Rhode Island's John Fogarty, who chaired the panel from the early 1950s until his death in 1967.

Flood was autocratic and rough, and very righteous—until 1979 when he resigned his chairmanship and later his seat in Congress because of his indictment for fraud. He was succeeded in the chair by William Natcher, a Kentuckian who was as dull as Flood was exciting, but who ran the subcommittee with an equally strong hand.

In the Senate, the chairmanship of the Appropriations subcommittee, after Hill, was held by Warren Magnuson, who later also became chairman of the full Appropriations Committee and the dean of the Senate. A passionate liberal who was usually very hard on his adversaries, Magnuson, at the age of 75, was retired from office in 1980 by his Washington constituents.

Whether a legislative proposal succeeds or fails in Congress is often as much a product of the talents, biases and interest of the chairmen of the subcommittees and committees in which it originates as it is of the soundness of the idea. This phenomenon is as apparent in the health area as in any other.

In the years immediately following World War II, when the federal government's reach was expanding in many ways as the country's resources and wealth grew dramatically, new health initiatives were largely limited to developing a strong and effective biomedical research program through the National Institutes of Health. Here is where John Fogarty and Lister Hill left their mark. Fogarty, a gruff bricklayer from Rhode Island who worked his subcommittee in a small room on the first floor of the Capitol to which no outsiders were admitted without invitation, each year started the process by writing the initial version of the NIH appropriations. Once the bill passed the House, Hill, the son of a noted Alabama physician, who was as urbane as Fogarty was gruff, picked up on the process in the Senate. The final product invariably carried a substantial increase. In 1955 the appropriation for NIH was $67 million; in 1960 it was $332 million; in 1965 it was $860 million; and in 1969, by which time both the House and Senate panels were under new leadership, the NIH appropriation had grown to $1.1 billion. The momentum kept up, propelled in part by high inflation, and in 1983 the appropriation for NIH was $4 billion. During this period the number of institutes grew from four to eleven. Fogarty and Hill have been justly credited with providing the primary impetus for developing the National Institutes of Health into an organization with the world's most preeminent biomedical research program. Without it, much of what else became a part of federal health policy would not have been possible.

When Hill and Fogarty were beginning to have their influence felt in the mid-1950s, the federal health effort consisted of little more than biomedical research and the level of funding for NIH was determined entirely by the appropriations process. The committees that had written the basic legislation setting up the institutes made the mandate very broad and general—it put no limitations on annual appropriations and did not require that the programs again be renewed by Congress by a certain date as most other authorizing legislation did.

But by the time a new generation of legislators assumed responsibility for health policy in the early 1970s, the situation had changed and the health subcommittees of the House Commerce Committee and the Senate Labor and Public Welfare Committee had a much more important role.

Paul Rogers was first on the scene as initially the de facto chairman and then the actual chairman of the Commerce health panel. Rogers, a dapper, even elegant man, was innately conservative, as appropriate to his Palm Beach, Florida, constituency, which from his first election in 1955 gave him an increasingly larger mandate every two years. In keeping with his conservative background, Rogers from his early days on the job had some serious reservations about the health programs his panel designed. He saw early a conglomeration of programs developing that often overlapped and even conflicted with one another. As chairman, he would seek to bring some order out of this apparent chaos. His style as a legislator was to work out a consensus before moving legislation to the floor. Rogers not only cultivated his fellow committee members, but anyone outside of Congress who worked on health issues—principals and staff in the Department of Health, Education and Welfare and lobbyists who coveted particular programs. His southern background made it easy for him to work closely with Republican members of his committee, and thus when he decided to go forward with a bill it was a good bet that he would be successful.

The legislation he developed generally was not broad or sweeping. Instead it would spotlight a problem—the need for more research in a particular area, lack of health care services to a certain category of people, the need for more physicians—and draft legislation designed to bring about some improvement. His bills kept those problems on a short rein—most would have to return in three years so the program managers could tell his committee how they were doing and what new resources they needed. He had no grand vision of what the federal responsibility in the health area should be; instead he worked at it piecemeal, dealing with problems as they came up.

Rogers was conservative, particularly in his early years as a health leader in Congress, but that conservatism eased somewhat in later years, and it never really applied to health programs. In 1970 he was given a low 24 percent rating as a legislator by the liberal Americans for Democratic Action and a high one of 68 percent by the Americans for Conservative Action. By 1976 his posture had changed and the ADA rated him 50 percent and the ACA 37 percent. Rogers never sponsored a national health insurance bill and said in an interview in 1983 that bringing about national health insurance in one fell swoop would not have been a good idea. If such a program were to come about, he said, it would be necessary to use an incremental approach, adding one feature at a time.[6] On the key vote in the Medicare debate on the House floor in 1965, Rogers voted against the program.

Edward Kennedy, who in 1971 became chairman of his health subcommittee, the Senate counterpart to Rogers's panel, was a sharp contrast to the Floridian. Born and raised in Boston, Kennedy was strongly imbued with the liberal Democratic ethic of the Boston Irish Catholic, and his political philosophy strongly resembled that of his two older brothers who had preceded him in national politics. Initially elected to the Senate two years after John Kennedy became president, Edward Kennedy showed no strong interest in health issues until the late 1960s. Although a member of the Labor and Public Welfare Committee since his first days in the Senate, he did not become a member of its health subcommittee until 1965, and by 1970 when Ralph Yarborough of Texas, then the panel's chairman, was preparing to leave office, Kennedy was still ranked fifth on the full committee. But by that time he had become interested in health issues and was able to persuade colleagues senior to him to let him have the chairmanship of the health panel. By that time also Kennedy had taken on the task of promoting national health insurance, and all of his work on the subcommittee revolved around this interest. Whatever legislation he considered, he sought to shape in a way that would build support for his national health insurance proposal. Thus Kennedy was always looking toward the day when Congress would enact a substantial new federal health responsibility, an approach that conflicted sharply with Rogers's shorter-range view of how the federal government should approach its health responsibilities. Nevertheless, the two found themselves working over the years to enact the same programs; the difference in their objectives for these programs would be more of size and scope than the services they were to provide.

Kennedy differed from Rogers in another important way. He started out proposing much more than he expected to get, expecting to compromise—and usually having to do so—as the bill worked its way through the legislative process. Kennedy worked with a much more liberal committee than Rogers, which made a difference, and thus by coincidence their styles suited well the initial legislative environment in which they worked. The difference between the two men could be most clearly seen in conference, where Rogers invariably knew the nitty-gritty details of the legislation substantially better than Kennedy. But in the end, Kennedy usually ended up with legislation pretty much as he had expected, and Rogers did too.

To the extent that there is a federal health policy, it is by and large defined by the government's financial support for health programs more than by what the goals of those programs, as expressed in their authorizing legislation, may be. That support is delineated in the official budget presented early each year to Congress by the president, and it is refined by Congress through its budget resolutions, appropriation bills and other legislation. The president's budget uses a somewhat arbitrary system to classify programs, and thus gives only a partial picture of federal health efforts. And even that picture is distorted. Most of the government's major health programs—Medicare, Medicaid and those run by the Public Health Service—are included in the health function, or section, of the budget. But this function also includes a number of minor programs—such as meat and poultry inspection and mine safety—that might more logically be included elsewhere in the federal budget structure. What is more, the health function excludes two of the major federal health programs—those operated by the Veterans Administration and the Department of Defense. It is through this incomplete prism that Congress and the Executive Branch view the country's health needs and seek to develop national health policy.

The distortion created by this budget arrangement is significant. When considering only the budget's health function, federal spending for health in fiscal 1983, the federal government's budget year that ended September 30, 1983, was an estimated $82.4 billion. But if the Defense Department and Veterans Administration health programs and the cost of the federal government's share of health insurance premiums for active and retired civil servants were included, the fiscal 1983 federal expenditures for health came to nearly $100 billion. And if revenue lost as result of tax deductions by individuals and business expenditures for health care were included, the total federal investment for health in fiscal 1983 was over $131 billion.[7]

The fact that Congress and the Executive Branch develop federal health policy through the distorted prism of the budget has broad ramifications, because it significantly underplays, by nearly 40 percent, the federal government's actual investment in the nation's health care system. More important, it suggests that the size of the leverage the federal government has over that system, by way of how it chooses to distribute this investment, is substantially less than is actually the case. This investment is in reality nearly half of all the more than $300 billion spent each year, from whatever source, on health care and related efforts in this country.

Through the Johnson administration, Congress relied heavily on the agencies of the Executive Branch for much of its staff work. He who controls the staff work controls to a large extent the final product, and so it was between Congress and the administration. Legislation was written in the Executive Branch, refined there, and the committee reports were largely written there. The end product was, thus, by and large what was wanted by the agency that would administer the program.

This relationship was largely developed in the New Deal days, the time when the federal government's role in relationship to society began to change substantially, and it was a relationship that grew and expanded through the years. Lyndon Johnson when he was pushing for enactment of his Great Society programs perfected the relationship; during those days Executive Branch personnel would shower congressional offices with documents, plans and legislative proposals. It was a relationship that would change in the early 1970s as Congress fought the contempt for it by the Nixon White House, a struggle for independence that reached its climax with the enactment of the 1974 Budget Control and Impoundment Act.

Specialized Health Programs Blossom

The demands on all levels of governments, but particularly on the federal government, to solve social problems are substantial, in both good times and bad. A reliance on the federal government to solve problems in the health area is perhaps greater than in other areas because some health issues can be solved only by government. Only government can ensure the safety of water supplies or quarantine contagious areas or people. Only the federal government can fully finance the tremendous biomedical research efforts underway in this country. Only the federal government can set standards for health services and care that are national in scope. And probably only the federal government can provide the financial support required to ensure that everyone in this country has full access to adequate health care.

Federal health programs as they are presented and shaped into legislative mandates are more often than not characterized by very high expectations. If it is the president who is proposing the program, he describes in glowing terms the good that would flow from it, in part to show that he is fulfilling his election mandate to make life better for Americans, and in part to begin to develop the necessary constituency that will be needed to help push the program through Congress. Once before Congress, the proposal picks up individual sponsors, whether because of an ideological commitment, out of loyalty to the president, a need to identify one's name with a desirable and beneficial program that will be received well by the voters once enacted, whether in response to pressure groups working through local constituencies, or, as is most likely, because of a combination of several or all of these forces.

Regardless of how momentum in support of the program builds, as the legislative process begins in earnest, some support inevitably is there, and it will be mobilized by the proposal's principal sponsors to help overcome opposition. Invariably, for health programs, that opposition does not deny a need for better health care—that would be like denying the need for motherhood. Instead, opponents argue that support for the program should come from other than the federal government.

For a health program to be successful, to overcome the opposition, which may be substantial, and to be enacted, the results that can be anticipated from its enactment are painted in ever more glowing terms. These heightened expectations are frequently accompanied by modifications in the original conceptual design of the program that the backers find necessary in order to win sufficient support to move the proposal along the legislative path to the president's desk.

Because of the tortuous path legislation must follow to become enacted, and because of the mixed feelings of most legislators about enacting substantial new programs in one large swoop, most domestic programs and certainly most health programs have been enacted in incremental stages. Rather than implanting a substantial new program all of a sudden on the health care system, Congress usually has chosen to create the program in increments—limited in scope at first, being expanded into a more comprehensive or definitive, and usually more expensive, program in subsequent legislative undertakings. This, of course, has kept members of Congress more involved in the program. They could monitor its development and more skillfully craft its expansion. They could also use the opportunity to demonstrate to their constituents concern for the sound fabric of the nation. Most health programs have been enacted incrementally, but not all. Some came into being fully conceptually, if not financially, developed, although changes in their design would be made as time went on.

Most of the specialized health programs created during the 1960s and 1970s generally were called categorical programs because they were designed to address a specific category of health care needs: community mental health centers to meet the lack of accessible mental health services, migrant health centers to provide health care to migrant farm workers who were not getting good care, family planning to help counter the problems created by unwanted pregnancies, and rat control to build a more healthy environment, for example. They were the spotlights used by Paul Rogers and Edward Kennedy to address health problems. While the categorical health programs have always accounted for only a small portion of the federal health bill, at most about $5 billion a year, they ultimately became the target of administration budget cutters because the amount spent on them could be controlled through the appropriations process. In this way they differed from Medicare and Medicaid where the federal government was obligated to pay for health services because of a person's age or disability, or because they were poor; for these programs the appropriation each year was a routine event.

Besides being directed at a particular need, the categorical programs enacted in the 1960s and early 1970s made federal funds available through grants for particular projects directly to community groups. In this way the federal programs jumped over the state and local governments that traditionally had responsibility for financing or nurturing local health care programs.

As new health problems arose or old ones acquired new urgency, the federal government would establish a new program or revamp an existing one to help deal with the problem. Those responsible for health policy in both the Executive Branch and Congress during this era believed, along with much of the public generally, the state and local governments were incapable of developing effective solutions on their own. Financial resources below the federal level were modest, as were those of personnel, both of professionals to deliver care and of the governmental bureaucracy to devise and carry out the programs. Thus, the federal government needed to be intimately involved, and the categorical health grant program became an increasingly popular device during the 1960s and the early 1970s for accomplishing this intimacy.

When such a program finally came into being, the results expected to flow from it, as vaguely perceived by the public, were then more often than not much greater than could realistically be expected. And since the proposal had a legislative life of only a few years, usually no more than three, very soon its managers again had to go before Congress to ask for new authority, a new level of appropriation authorization and changes in the basic program to make it work better and respond to new demands. In this process, Congress often changed direction, sometimes confusing those in the field who ran the programs or were its beneficiaries.

The tremendous expansion of federal involvement in financing and providing health care that began in the 1960s was in response to a universally recognized need for more and better health care for the American people, a need that could only be met if the federal government got involved. No other level of government, no number or combination of private agencies could do the job without substantial federal involvement.

But there was ambivalence from the start. While liberal and conservative politicians divided along traditional lines over to what extent the federal government should be involved in financing and delivering health care, even those who supported the initial thrust soon began to realize that the extent of federal involvement was becoming unwieldy, and in the process causing many problems, and sometimes more than they solved.

Paul Rogers, who in 1971 became chairman of the House Commerce health subcommittee, in 1966 was already a leader in the House on health issues and that year he chaired a special panel to examine health programs of the Department of Health, Education and Welfare. The report of that study, published in October, argued that the emerging conglomeration of specialized programs designed to develop federal, state and local partnerships to meet existing problems was seriously fragmented, and as a result agencies at the different levels of government were "forced to go shopping in the 'federal market' for various bits and pieces of an overall health program."[8] The report went on:

> The subcommittee was impressed with the fact that the great mass of legislation, regulations, and interpretations of regulations, characterizing the HEW health-related financial assistance programs proved to be so complex and multifaceted as to confuse not only the health authorities at the state and local levels but even officials within the department itself. . . . Some grant-in-aid programs require matching funds while others do not. Among those requiring matching funds, the percentages required are not uniform. Some require prior approval of the grant application by the appropriate state authority while others have no such requirement. There also exists a diversity of forms which must be employed in applying for the various grants.[9]

The report recommended an increased emphasis on comprehensive support for health services and at the same time a deemphasis on categorical grants as a device to support health services. In the panel's view, "project and categorical funds insofar as they are applied to existing health services programs have substantially served their original purpose of stimulation. They appear to be unsuitable for the primary need of the present time, i.e. the need for a firm base of coordinated federal support" to states for comprehensive health care. The need for "federal stimulation is past and what is needed now is a continuing support for comprehensive general health programs," the report concluded.[10]

This was in 1966 when many, but by no means all, the categorical health grant programs had been enacted. Congress did not heed the committee's advice, except for some consolidation of general Public Health Service authority. Indeed, Rogers himself, as he led the health subcommittee, pushed for the enactment of more specialized, or categorical, health grant programs.

There were other congressional expressions of concern over the way the federal government's role in health was developing. A 1970 study by the Senate Government Operations Committee found that federal health programs "comprise a cumbersome, disjointed bureaucracy that key government officials have difficulty managing."[11] The uncoordinated proliferation of health programs, the panel's report said, results in a situation in which agencies whose priorities are not related to health make decisions that affect people's health. It also found "little evidence of any general effort to use federal health dollars as a lever for changing and improving the nation's health care system. . . . Each program and each agency was an island unto itself. Each program and each agency's involvement in health may have occurred as a necessary response to a certain problem. But when viewed in combinations or as a whole, both programs and agency health missions . . . appeared to have little relationship to each other or the health needs of the American people."[12] As a result, the panel's report concluded:

> Federal programs have not attempted to come to grips with rising health care costs. Federal programs have only touched on the problem of limited access to care. Federal programs have not tried to pull together, or provide incentives, to develop models of organized delivery systems for the general population. Federal programs have been woefully inadequate in dealing with the shortage and distribution of health manpower. . . . The extensive fragmentation of federal health programs makes it difficult to consider broad issues in coherent manner . . . [and as a result] federal health programs touch on every problem of health care delivery without dealing decisively with any one.[13]

Some effort was made by Congress to respond to this concern by building a health planning system, an effort that was actually begun right after World War II. In 1946 Congress enacted the Hill-Burton hospital construction program, which ultimately was responsible for building thousands of hospitals providing for nearly a half-million beds throughout the country, many in rural areas that were, by 1946, very short on health facilities. In fact, the program, generally viewed as a major plus in the nation's arsenal of health legislation, was responsible for cementing into the health care system a strong bias toward inpatient, and thus by the 1980s expensive, care, although when the program was launched hospitals were much more necessary to treat most illnesses than they are today.

The Hill-Burton program, however, was not just a hospital construction program. It contemplated that states would see that those hospitals were built in accordance with some sort of overall plan. A variety of legislation was enacted during the early 1960s, some amending Hill-Burton and some creating new authority, expanding the federal role in health planning. By 1966 the array of federal grants for planning and for the support of services had become complex and intertwined.

In 1966, Congress enacted the comprehensive health planning act that among other things consolidated some of the fragmented authorities for funding health services. But no sooner had this partial consolidation taken place than more new and separate specialized health programs were enacted.

The community mental health centers (CMHC) program was one of the categorical grant programs that got started in the early 1960s and grew substantially over the next decade and a half. It was a scheme of federal grants to communities and state and local governments to support the delivery of mental health services on an outpatient basis. Most categorical programs developed incrementally, rising from modest pilot or demonstration programs to full-fledged, substantial, semipermanent grant-in-aid efforts as a result of periodic renewals and expansions. In contrast, the CMHC program sprouted nearly full-blown onto the health care arena.

The federal government had had very little to do with providing mental health services until the 1960s. The first effort toward this end occurred over 100 years earlier when Congress in 1854 passed legislation, the idea for which had been proposed by Dorothea Dix, setting aside more than 12 million acres of federal land for facilities to provide treatment for the indigent and insane. That proposal was vetoed by President Franklin Pierce on the grounds that it would usurp the responsibilities of states. Over the next century, the state asylum system grew, and the belief that the mentally ill should be isolated from the rest of society grew along with it.[14]

During World War II the state system deteriorated dramatically. Professional and support personnel were drafted to aid the war effort, and both patients and facilities were neglected. By the end of the war, many mentally ill patients in state hospitals were living in horrible conditions. The end of the war, however, brought back into civilian practice a number of people who had begun to believe that the mentally ill could be better cared for if they continued to live and work in their communities while receiving treatment.

In response to this new concern, in 1946 the National Institute of Mental Health (NIMH) was created as part of the National Institutes of

Health. The new institute focused on research and training, but some federal aid was authorized for grants to states for prevention and treatment of mental illness.

Once formed, NIMH, under the leadership for nearly the next twenty years of its first director, Robert Felix, a psychiatrist, became the spawning ground for a new concept in the delivery of health care—a system of comprehensive care that sought to ensure that everyone living within a specific geographic area received the care they needed in one facility, regardless of their ability to pay. It was also an effort to have the treatment of mental illness and psychiatric disorders viewed as physical disabilities were viewed—problems that could generally be solved, or at least alleviated. Through the years, psychiatric problems had carried a social stigma and as a result were ostracized by the main stream of medicine. Among other things, the CMHC program helped to mitigate that attitude.

The comprehensive care concept was to become very important in the debate over how health care services generally, not just mental health services, should be organized. It was in this case a concept articulated in the recommendations of the Joint Commission on Mental Illness and Health created by Congress in 1955. Six years later, in 1961, the commission filed its final report after producing what was, until that time, the most comprehensive review and analysis of mental health care in the country. The principal recommendation of the commission called for the creation of community mental health clinics to be operated as outpatient departments of general or mental hospitals, as part of state or regional health care systems, or as independent agencies. That recommendation was turned into a legislative proposal and pushed by President Kennedy. Rather than providing for the gradual evolution of a new federal program through demonstration programs and pilot projects, the measure called for the creation of an entirely new system of mental health care that when completed would leave a mental health center in every community in the country. It was largely due to President Kennedy's support and the spade work by the original advocates of the program in educating Congress to the desirability of enacting the progam in one fell swoop that it was able to hurdle the incremental step.

Two kinds of federal grants under the program were to be made to local and state governments and private nonprofit community agencies. The first followed a well-established formula by providing funds for the construction of mental health facilities in communities throughout the country. The second, however, proposed something radically new. It would provide funds for paying psychiatrists as well as other mental health professionals and support personnel to staff the centers. These grants would be phased out over a period of about four years, at which time local governments or the communities would be expected to provide the resources to continue funding the program. Never before had the federal government provided dollars to hire physicians to deliver care, unless they were actually federal employees.

In 1963, subcommittees in both the House and Senate reviewed the proposal as sent forward by the administration and approved it. The Senate version went on to win approval by the full committee and later by the full Senate, but opposition had developed by the time that version came to the House.

The American Medical Association had expressed no objection to the staffing grant when the legislation was first proposed, probably because it simply overlooked its implications. But by the time the proposal had passed the Senate and was ready to be considered by the full House Interstate and Foreign Commerce Committee, the AMA had given the matter more thought; it now officially opposed the measure. The more conservative members of the organization saw the staffing grant as the first step in a scheme of socialized medicine, one in which all physicians ultimately would become employees of the federal government. This, of course, was at the time the AMA was fighting, successfully, enactment of Medicare. The medical profession's opposition was enough to defeat the proposal. The House panel rejected the staffing grant, accepting only the construction grant, and that version was the one that finally cleared Congress and was signed by President Kennedy in October 1963, a month before his death.

The staffing grant, however, was to be enacted two years later, in 1965, after Lyndon Johnson won the presidency in his own right and had a substantial majority in Congress to back him up. By that time, the AMA was enmeshed in its losing struggle to prevent Medicare's enactment, and so it abandoned its concern over the now relatively minor mental health centers staffing program.

Once both parts of the community mental health centers program—construction and staffing—were enacted, subsequent changes were to be incremental. At first these changes would enhance the comprehensive concept of the program, and then ultimately tear it apart.

The concept of the comprehensive care system embedded in the CMHC act was to become one of the most important in the debate over how health care services generally should be organized. It meant, in the case of mental health centers, that a person could receive whatever kind of care he might need through one program. Medical records would be available to all those delivering care to the individual, and often all the care necessary—outpatient, inpatient, etc.—would be provided under the same roof. If the program did not have an inpatient unit in its principal facility, it used beds in a nearby hospital and its personnel would be involved in the treatment program there. Continuity of care was emphasized. Later, this same concept would become central to the health maintenance organization program as well as to the debate over national health insurance. The purists in the NHI debate, such as

Edward Kennedy, maintained that a system of health care, where treatment of one kind was linked to another, was crucial not only to the best kind of health care but also to paring the cost of care.

Further, the mental health center sought to reach beyond its doors to help the community generally create a more healthy psychological environment. The center worked on the traditional public health basis; it was responsible for a specific geographic area—called a catchment area—that was determined by population, normally between 50,000 and 200,000. The center was to be the guardian of the mental health of all those who lived in the catchment area, although no one would be required to use its services if they chose not to. Those who did use its services would pay according to their ability to do so. Through the center's consultation and education program, mental health professionals worked with schools, factories, businesses and other social or economic entities to create a more healthy environment.

The CMHC program became very popular on Capitol Hill. Mental health centers were built in communities all over the country, frequently with a senator's or congressman's name on the door. Moreover, they were generally well received by those communities, an enthusiasm that got back to the people in Congress. From 1963 through 1978, the program was always given new and expanded authority, and several times during this fifteen-year period it was the fair-haired child that provided the vehicle for renewing authority for other programs. But its short life was nevertheless topsy-turvy. Extended or expanded into the 1970s, it was first embraced by President Nixon and then attacked. Its next phase was to take on, along with other health programs, the Nixon administration as it attempted to impound funds.

One federal health effort that largely fulfilled its goals, and thus faded from the scene because it had done so, was the program to train more health care personnel, primarily doctors. It was able to do so in part because the training programs were well funded, but also because it differed fundamentally from other health programs; it was a program to stimulate production of a product, the physician—not to provide a service.

While the supply of physicians and other health care personnel was a serious problem, the proper role of the federal government in helping to train doctors and other health care practitioners was a major element in the debate over national health policy, a debate that lasted for nearly two decades. The issues were complex because of the length of time training often takes, constructing a federal training policy required projections of changes in the population, the likely resulting changes in demands on the nation's health care system, and the number of physicians to be graduated each year.

Rationale for federal intervention in the health care sector is invariably based on the need to correct an imbalance or provide a stimulus that otherwise would not arise. But once the intervention is made, once the federal support has begun, what follows is an increasingly complex set of arrangements of supports, and further supports to correct imbalances created by the initial program or to preserve the initial investment. Those who are the immediate beneficiaries of federal support create their own systems to ensure that the program is enhanced rather than depleted. Whatever the real needs of the nation, it eventually becomes extremely difficult for the federal government to extricate itself from the arrangement it has created. The switch may cause such substantial disruption in one quarter or another that it becomes a politically risky undertaking. Although the change in policy may be made, it is seldom made swiftly and almost never without agony.

So it was with the history of federal support for training health care personnel.

During the sixties and seventies, the federal government invested more than $3 billion in training health care professionals, much of it for training physicians. While medical schools welcomed federal support from the first, the American Medical Association was initially reluctant; only comparatively recently did it come to endorse it. AMA reluctance was grounded in traditional apprehension over federal interference in the private relationship between doctor and patient, and in apprehension over how the federal government might try to control the medical profession. If the federal government paid for all or a significant portion of the cost of educating a doctor, the AMA reasoned, it might, too, seek to control how and where the young physician practiced medicine.

The spectrum of health care professionals recognized in federal legislation was broad. It ranged from doctors of medicine and osteopathy, to nurses and podiatrists, to physician assistants, and to public health personnel whose job it is to treat the environment rather than the individual. Even veterinarians for years were included in the package of health care personnel offered training support by the federal government. But physicians are the hub of the nation's health care delivery system and thus the central focus of the federal training program.

Substantial federal support for medical education began in the early 1960s, after federal health policy-makers became convinced that the country would soon experience a shortage of health care personnel, particularly physicians, unless steps were taken to stimulate the medical educational system. They also, at that time, recognized that aggravated shortages existed in areas where setting up practice was least desirable—in rural communities and city ghettos.

The initial programs of support—very modest ones—began two decades earlier. Federal dollars began to flow to biomedical research programs in the early 1940s. For the next twenty years this was the principal way the federal government had of supporting the nation's medical education system. Federal funds went to research facilities with few strings attached. The mandate was broad. Then, as later, much of the federal support for research was used to pay the salaries of researchers—trained physicians who had chosen to work in the laboratory rather than in the consulting room. These research funds also went to employ those in other disciplines—Ph.D.'s in a variety of fields—who also pursued careers in biomedical research. But as these institutions developed their own training programs, they began to use some of the federal funds to support those being trained as researchers.

Support for research training was in keeping with the substantial federal investment being made in biomedical research itself. The investment helped research institutions become the dominant entity in the medical arena and, thus, the guts of the medical training system.

Then, during World War II, when the military services found that there were not enough doctors in the civilian population to meet their needs, programs were created to speed the training of doctors and to train more of them. Once the war was over, federal support subsided. But the major federal health training programs really began in 1963.

That year, federal policy-makers, confronted with data showing a rapidly expanding population, became persuaded that a doctor shortage was on the horizon. Both the administration and Congress dominated by Democrats agreed that the federal government should accept responsibility for stimulating the training of greater numbers of physicians. The legislation enacted that year authorized grants for constructing or expanding medical school facilities and providing loans to students, arguing that not to do so would result in a waste of earlier federal investments.

The report of the House committee that fashioned this legislation noted that existing federal programs had stimulated construction of hospitals and other health care facilities. Without federal support for training, it said, these investments would be jeopardized and the original grants would have to be cut off because the new facilities could not be used.[15] Also a number of studies urged immediate increase in the number of physicians. In 1950 there had been a ratio of one general practitioner for each 1,300 people, but by 1960 there was only one doctor for each 1,700 people. The gap was expected to continue to widen; by 1975 there would only be one doctor for each 2,000 people unless more physicians were trained.[16] Past expenditure of federal funds now required an even greater expenditure.

The 1963 law was also designed in part to encourage newly graduated physicians to practice in remote areas where doctors were scarce, thus attempting to deal with what turned out to be the most intractable aspect of federal training policy. Up to half of the education debt would be waived if the borrower practiced in parts of the country where physicians were in short supply.

Federal support for training physicians and other health care personnel expanded during the 1960s and into the 1970s, but then, as with other federal health efforts, a dichotomy developed. The training programs were costing more and more, a burden that became increasingly aggravating as the flush financial times of the 1960s faded into the hard times of the 1970s. As the impact of the programs increased and increasingly bothered some whom they touched, the luster diminished. Opposition both within and without the federal government developed.

By 1983, federal programs supporting health training had been largely dismantled, and with a surplus of doctors on the horizon the remaining problems—a shortage of doctors in rural and poor areas and a shortage of primary care physicians, or general practitioners—seemed to be on the verge of solution.

Because of the developing surplus, and thus the competition for business, young doctors, on their own volition, were establishing practices in out-of-the-way places that had no doctor, or had a serious shortage of them. And because there was more need for the general practitioner, more were offering this service instead of pursuing careers as specialists. In addition, fees doctors were charging were moderating, or at least not climbing as fast. The federal investment had paid off.

Reservations by various members and committees of Congress, of all political stripes, about the role of the federal government in the nation's health care system were to continue through the seventies. When President Ford in 1975 and again in 1976 proposed converting a number of health programs into block grants—federal funding that would go to the states with few strings attached—he was turned down by Congress, but even then there clearly was sentiment for the change; the opposition was almost entirely political, for a presidential campaign was on the horizon and Congress, controlled by Democrats, was not at this point going to adopt such a dramatic reversal in policy proposed by a Republican president. Not until President Reagan entered the White House in 1981 with sufficient political muscle behind him would Congress go along with the shift in philosophy.

Medicare Is Born

In the midst of the ferment and mushrooming of federally supported health programs at the beginning of Lyndon Johnson's Great Society era, Medicare and, almost as an afterthought, Medicaid in 1965 were enacted. This was one of that era's major accomplishments and a major event in the history of federal health policy for a number of reasons. In one sense Medicare was a national health insurance program for the elderly, and many thought it would lay the groundwork for universal health care coverage. If nothing else, the age of entry, 65, could be lowered in subsequent amendments, following the traditional incremental approach to enacting domestic programs. Indeed, just such changes would be made. In 1972, Medicare would be opened to the disabled and those with chronic kidney disease.

But what was not anticipated was that the costs of Medicare and Medicaid would rise so dramatically; as a result the programs became the principal barrier to passage of a more comprehensive program. Over the years, health care costs had risen in tandem with wages, and since federal health policy-makers expected that pattern to continue, any rise in health care costs would be accommodated by higher revenues from payroll taxes due to increased wages. That pattern, however, did not continue to hold, and health care costs started rising at a greater clip than wages. By 1983, Medicare and Medicaid were hugh efforts costing together $76.7 billion a year.[17] Because of their costs, Medicare and Medicaid dominated federal health policy since their enactment and would continue to do so as long as there was no federal health program that cost more.

By 1965, the forces that had opposed the enactment of Medicare had been somewhat dissipated. President Johnson's victory in 1964 with 61 percent of the vote was sufficiently strong to put on the defensive the American Medical Association and its colleagues in the medical world who had been over the years the principal opponents of Medicare. Johnson's victory also weakened the conservative coalition of Republicans and southern Democrats that had dominated Congress during the postwar years and that in 1963 had lost one of its principal members when Robert Kerr, who along with Wilbur Mills had been responsible for enactment in 1960 of Kerr-Mills, died.

Although both the House and Senate were already controlled by Democrats, that party's majority increased in each as a result of the 1964 elections. In the Senate where, as noted, there had already been enough strength to pass the administration's Medicare program, the Democratic majority rose in 1965 by two members, to 68. In the House, 38 seats switched parties, raising the Democratic total to 295, more than a two-to-one majority. Indeed, the 38-member increase for the Democrats was more than it appeared, for among the new members were 42 northern Democrats, all supporters of Medicare. It would not only be enough to pass Medicare once it got to the floor, but the change was sufficient to persuade Wilbur Mills, the principal roadblock in the House, that he should join the effort.

Medicare and Medicaid are two very different programs with different objectives, different financing schemes and to some extent different origins. By and large, too, the people they serve are different, although some receive benefits under both programs. But they were enacted at the same time, and as a result have usually been viewed together. When changes were considered, they were pushed forward in a Medicare-Medicaid package.

The two programs work quite differently. Medicare is an insurance program in which the federal government acts as the insurance company and regular insurance companies act as the agent, or the intermediary, paying bills for the government. The program is financed in several ways: in part by payroll taxes on both employees and employers, in part by premiums paid by the beneficiaries and in part by contributions from the general revenues of the U.S. Treasury.

There are two separate Medicare programs, part A, which covers institutional care, primarily hospitals, and part B, which pays for care by doctors. In 1983, everyone who was a social security beneficiary was automatically eligible for part A Medicare insurance, and that included almost everyone 65 years of age or older, plus the disabled and persons with chronic kidney failure—a total of 29.7 million people. This group could participate in part B by paying a monthly premium. Those elderly not included were largely former government personnel, and even they could buy into the program by purchasing coverage, although in most cases they had their own health insurance and thus did not elect to join Medicare.

Medicare beneficiaries when using hospital services (part A) must pay for the first day of care (about $350 in 1983). The cost of care for the second through the sixtieth day of hospitalization is fully covered, and from the sixty-first through the ninetieth day the beneficiary pays 25 percent of the cost. From the ninety-first day through the one hundred and fiftieth, he pays 50 percent of the cost, and after that all charges. When outpatient services and physician care (whether in the hospital or out of it) are used, Medicare, after an initial deductible (applied each year), pays 80 percent of the cost that it allows for that service. The patient must pay at least 20 percent of the bill, and perhaps more if the fee charged by the physician is more than allowed by Medicare.

There is an important distinction between the two parts of Medicare, however, beyond cost-sharing for the beneficiary. Hospitals are prohibited by law from charging the beneficiary more than Medicare allows for the care, except for the initial deductible for the first day of care and copayments beyond the sixtieth day of hospitalization. A physician, on the other hand, can charge the patient the difference between what Medicare allows for the service and what the physician normally charges.

Medicaid, in contrast to Medicare, is a grant program in which the federal government shares with states the cost of health care services received by certain welfare recipients. States run the program pursuant to federal guidelines, paying directly those who provide the care. These providers are not allowed to charge the patient an additional amount, as a physician treating a Medicare beneficiary can, and patients are not generally reimbursed for care for which they have paid, as often happens under Medicare.

States were required to provide certain basic services (such as hospital care) as part of their Medicaid programs and could choose to provide certain supplementary services (such as paying for eyeglasses). Payment for services, although actually made by the state, was patterned after the fee-for-service principle embedded in the Medicare program. The federal share of the cost of each state's Medicaid program was between 50 percent and 83 percent. Where the person was 65 or older as well as poor, he or she also received Medicare coverage.

Medicaid, which replaced the 1960 Kerr-Mills program and several other health care programs designed to help the poor, became the primary device by which the federal government sought to ensure that the poor got adequate medical care. There were a number of other programs—such as community health centers and migrant health centers that complemented this effort—but Medicaid was the centerpiece from which just about all health care to the poor flowed.

Because Medicaid was primarily a state program and benefits varied widely from state to state, poor people were given different levels of medical care simply because of where in the country they lived.

Through the early 1980s, debates over extending the federal government's role in financing health care focused on the need to "reform" the system, which meant changing the way providers, or those who deliver care, were paid. Traditionally, physicians were paid a fee specified by the doctor for a specific service—a physical exam, a hospital visit, a flu shot. The hospital, working much the same way, established specific charges for its services—a day in bed, this test, or that. Because there were no limits—except those set by competition for patients in the health care marketplace—on how high the doctor fee or hospital charge might go, the patient had to pay pretty much what the doctor or hospital billed. When Medicare was being considered, that tradition did not seem to be a serious problem, for health care costs were rising at that time only moderately, although fast enough to become a worrisome burden for the elderly. Thus, those drafting the legislation made no effort to "reform" the payment system and instead pledged the federal government under Medicare to pay whatever the doctor billed, provided it was the usual and customary charge in the area for that service. The hospital was to be reimbursed for its cost in providing care. The provision was not a compromise on the part of the bill's sponsors to gain the support of the medical profession; even with this provision, the AMA was adamantly opposed to the legislation. Instead, the government, both as represented by members of Congress and officials in the Executive Branch, was proposing that the practice followed in private industry between insurance companies and hospitals be used by this new government program.

With the federal government, once Medicare came into being, paying for much of the cost of care for the elderly, these costs began to rise significantly, and there was no way the bill payer, the federal government, could easily check that rise. The frustration was aggravated by the fact that hospitals and doctors in different parts of the country would charge different amounts for the same care. Thus, politicians and federal health policy-makers became reluctant to expand the federal commitment without also adopting a device that protected the federal government against high inflation in health care prices—and this protective device was elusive and hard to define. Reforms of the system, regardless of who sat in the White House, when one got down to the nuts and bolts of it, generally focused on ways of setting specific limits on what the federal government would pay for a particular service—in other words, federal regulation.

With Lyndon Johnson's victory and the demise of the conservative coalition, Wilbur Mills realized that he would have to compromise and accept the enactment of some sort of health legislation with the social security mechanism. Mills in an interview in 1983 talked about this switch. He maintained that favorable consideration of legislation of the magnitude of Medicare is a matter of timing. He had not supported it in earlier years, he suggested, because he could not put together the coalition necessary to win its enactment. Now, with Johnson's victory and the new Democratic strength in the House, he could. He was ready to move, and he wanted to move and to help Johnson enact his program, he said, in the 1983 interview. With this change, the way was cleared for Medicare.

Other forces also gathered in 1965 to provide substantial support for its enactment. Costs of hospital care were going up faster than other costs, and increasingly the need was felt to provide protection for the poor and the aged against the possibility of medical bills that could use up all their savings.

With his new mandate behind him, Johnson did not want to miss his chance, and despite this mandate he knew that he might miss it if he waited too long. So he pushed House and Senate Democratic leaders to move quickly, and they accommodated this request; early consideration was scheduled.

The original administration Medicare proposal was, in fact, quite modest, much more modest than the ultimate product. The Johnson bill, like the King-Anderson bill before it, covered only the costs of hospitalization, skilled nursing home care for recuperation and home health services after hospitalization, and certain outpatient diagnostic services. The bill as finally enacted also covered a portion of the cost of most physician fees and outpatient care.

The metamorphosis occurred in the Ways and Means Committee where all taxing legislation, by tradition, starts. Early in 1965 Johnson sent his Medicare proposal to Congress; Mills was now ready to get action on it. John Byrnes, then the ranking Republican member, proposed an alternative that would have the federal government pay a portion of the cost of all medical care—both hospital and physician services—for the elderly, but unlike the administration's program, participation in this would be voluntary. The Byrnes bill had its origin in a measure backed by the American Medical Association, but under that proposal states would have been required to sponsor the program. The administration's program covering hospital costs was to be paid for entirely by an increase in the social security tax earmarked for Medicare; but the Byrnes proposal would be financed differently—by a separate premium to be paid for in part by the beneficiary and in part by the federal government through contributions from general revenues of the Treasury. Again, as in 1950, the payment scheme was to be an important distinction.

Mills was strongly in favor of the payroll tax as a device to finance Medicare, but Byrnes was just as equally opposed to it, and in the end even though his voluntary program covering outpatient care was part of the proposal, Byrnes and the other GOP members of the panel opposed the bill. Byrnes argued that the payroll tax approach was a poor concept upon which to base the program because, as he told the House during its debate on the measure, to do so was to sell the program on the understanding that by participating in it beneficiaries would have certain levels of care coming to them as a right. Under such a concept, he said, there would be "no flexibility to make changes because the people tell you, 'We have bought this and you cannot make any change except to liberalize it.' " Mills argued that a payroll tax would tend to "limit the growth of the benefit and will tend to do so to a greater extent" than if the costs are paid for out of the general funds of the Treasury.[18]

Mills's implied argument that in order to increase benefits you would have to increase the tax was correct and, in fact, the tax has been increased steadily over the years as program costs have increased, even though, on balance, benefits have been depleted. But Byrnes perhaps saw more accurately the dilemma for the future. Medicare and Medicaid have together, over the years of their existence, gotten the lion's share of the federal government's increased contribution to health care. Medicare and Medicaid have gone on growing unchecked by the usual congressional appropriations process, and the only way to get control has been to enact legislation changing the basic authority of the program, a procedure that generally has been very difficult to pursue because of the resistance in Congress to denying people a benefit they already had.

Although some paring of Medicare benefits occurred over the years, cutbacks in the cost of the program came about largely as a result of putting caps on what providers could charge. By 1983, however, the Reagan administration had largely exhausted the possibility of savings through this approach and was considering making the Medicare beneficiary pay more for the cost of his health care—and it was facing terrific opposition, just as Byrnes had predicted.

When it came time in the early spring of 1965 for the Ways and Means Committee to vote on the bill, Mills offered not only the administration's package, but Byrnes's package covering outpatient and physician services, thus substantially expanding the initial administration proposal.

Mills later woud say this was necessary to gain sufficient support for the program and to be fair to the beneficiary, for the administration's plan would have only covered 25 percent of an elderly person's health care costs.[19]

At the same time, Mills, in a surprise move, proposed broadening the existing Kerr-Mills program to cover most people, regardless of age, on welfare, and those with low incomes who would be moved onto welfare because of their health care costs. Like Kerr-Mills, this new program—Medicaid—would be up to the state to administer. The federal government would pay about half the cost and set minimal standards for services. This combination became known as the three-layered cake—full health care coverage for the poor, guaranteed hospital insurance for the elderly, and payment of outpatient and physician costs for the elderly who chose it.

When Mills's committee reported the Medicare bill on March 29, 1965, by a straight party-line 17–8 vote, all Democrats, including Mills, voted for the measure. The previous year the administration's plan had been able to draw only twelve votes in favor, and Mills had not been among them. When the measure got to the floor, on the crucial vote, which was a Republican motion to send it back to committee, or recommit it, the Democratic position prevailed 236 to 191;[20] the 42 new liberal Democrats elected in 1964 were what was needed. Since the margin of victory on this key vote was 45 votes, a switch of 23 would have defeated the measure.

Mills, of course, by going along in 1965, avoided being on the losing side, but, more important, he positioned himself to have a dominant say in shaping the new program, not only that year but in later years. The final version of the measure was mostly the House bill, and contained little of what the Senate had added.

The Republican members of the Ways and Means Committee, in their minority report, said they fully supported the "concept that adequate health insurance should be made available to the aged at a reasonable cost,"[21] but with equal fervor they rejected the mandatory hospital insurance program that was the core of the Democratic proposal.

Furthermore, they argued that any funds contributed by the federal government should be paid out of the general funds of the Treasury rather than derived from a payroll tax. The payroll tax was regressive, they argued, since it taxed everyone at the same rate with the result that the burden fell most heavily on the poor. Using the payroll tax to finance Medicare would undermine the program and threaten cash benefits for retirement. Furthermore, unlike the retirement program, costs of the Medicare program would be impossible to predict, and they were right. The costs of Medicare in the early years of the program were wholly unpredictable.

If the GOP minority, led by Byrnes, was prescient in this regard, it also accurately anticipated another serious problem—a phenomenon that has become known as cost shift. Medicare, the Republicans said, was not going to pay the full cost of hospital services for the elderly because payment would be based on reasonable costs rather than on the customary charge that the hospital generally levied. Reasonable cost was to be determined by Medicare's administrators, and could be anything these administrators determined, the Republicans suggested. In fact, adjustments in reasonable costs have been the principal way Medicare costs have been scaled back in recent years. "If hospitals are prevented from charging the customary rates to the patients over 65, hospital costs for patients under age 65 will have to be increased in order to make up the difference," the GOP minority report said.[22] In 1979, this cost shift amounted to $3 billion. In 1982, it was $6 billion.[23]

Three and a half years after Medicare and Medicaid began operating, a study by the Senate Finance Committee found the programs were "in serious financial trouble . . . [and] adversely affecting health care costs and financing for the general population." Unless, the report went on, "the rapid and continuing escalation in the costs of health care are moderated, the Congress may reasonably anticipate increasing pressure upon it to extend the . . . programs to encompass large segments of the population not now covered under these public health payment plans."[24]

As Medicare and Medicaid provided less and less coverage, they became increasingly the butt of criticism. Although when it first began in 1966, Medicare paid, on the average, 50 percent of the total cost of the annual health care bill of an elderly person, by 1980 it covered only about 40 percent.[25] The reductions were accomplished primarily through enactment of legislation placing further limits on benefits and by physician fees rising faster than compensatory payments by Medicare. But for many elderly, those who did not require extensive nursing care, the statistics were misleading. Nursing care was the major health care cost of those who needed it, and Medicare paid relatively little of the overall nursing care bill for the elderly. Those elderly who did not require nursing care—only hospital and physician care—would have a substantial portion of their health care costs covered by Medicare.

The House Aging Committee, after a prolonged study, in 1980 concluded that Medicare, although a highly successful program in many regards, was under stress and at risk of substantial deterioration. Beneficiaries were becoming increasingly disillusioned with the program because the extent of coverage was continually diminishing. Each year the elderly were being required to pay more out of their own pockets to participate in Medicare, and as a result they were finding it increasingly necessary to purchase supplemental health insurance to pick up where Medicare left off. There were a lot of gaps in Medicare coverage. Eyeglasses, dental care, outpatient drugs, hearing aids, as well as most nursing home care were not covered, for example. The program had been further warped by the fact that a large portion of Medicare funds went to pay for services to relatively few beneficiaries with large medical bills.

Medicare and Medicaid were criticized because they provided only partial, not total, health care for the elderly and poor, and particularly because they did not protect them from the catastrophic costs of severe illnesses. Furthermore, because the traditional health care system was geared toward institutional care, most of the money spent through Medicare and Medicaid on the elderly and the poor was spent for the kind of care that very often was not the most advantageous to the beneficiary—there was no emphasis on care designed to prevent the development of illness or infirmity.

Thus, Medicare became more and more a disappointment for its beneficiaries, and as a result the caution with which politicians approached national health insurance increased out of concern that it, too, would be simply another program of failed expectations.

It is part of the irony of the history of national health insurance that the two federal programs—Medicare and Medicaid, which many saw as the forerunner of NHI—have instead made the country generally, and lawmakers particularly, apprehensive about launching a new massive federal health care effort. Initially modest programs with anticipated expenses in 1967 of about $4 billion, Medicare and Medicaid had by 1983 grown to a level where together their combined costs were rising each year by $9 billion, more than twice the amount of the estimated total annual initial cost of the program.

2
THE MIDDLE YEARS

The problem of increasingly expensive Medicare and Medicaid programs was compounded by the fact that neither was designed to change in any way the existing health care system and its financing mechanisms. Indeed, services delivered through these programs were to be paid for in the traditional way—a fee for a service in the case of physician care; reimbursement of cost in the case of hospital care. There was nothing in Medicare and Medicaid that supported, or even encouraged, more efficient and effective ways of delivering health care. As a result, neither could be used creatively to support new organizational forms of health care delivery, such as neighborhood health centers, health maintenance organizations or community mental health centers. Such programs were going to have to get their federal funds from the regular appropriations process, and in fact, in one sense, would have to compete with Medicare and Medicaid for increasingly scarce health care dollars.

What is more, the strong bias in Medicare and Medicaid for the use of the traditional systems of health care meant that alternative ways of providing services were not able to get a secure foothold. Categorical grant programs, representing the new ways of providing care and that ultimately might have been able to provide the leverage necessary to change the way health care services were delivered, were, as a practical matter, relegated to a back seat. Many believed, for example, that community health centers—begun as part of the poverty program and designed to provide care primarily to the poor—had the potential for delivering health care more efficiently than the traditional private market, but significant increases in federal support for these programs or other systems of care was not forthcoming.

These categorical programs each year had to get their spending money through the regular appropriations process, and every few years new authorizing legislation had to be enacted. In contrast, Medicare and Medicaid, because they required neither new authorization periodically nor annual appropriations—the original act provided funds would automatically flow to them in amounts necessary to pay for the cost of care that their beneficiaries received—were able to grow fully in response to demand. Some members of the committees that authorized the categorical programs expected that at some point Medicare and Medicaid would be opened up in a way that would allow those dollars to be used to pay for services provided by community health centers or mental health centers, for example. Those who sat on the Finance and Ways and Means committees may have initially thought, as well, this might happen, but as Medicare and Medicaid grew, and grew so big so quickly, beyond what its authors had expected, they became very apprehensive about opening up these programs in any way that might increase their costs. So the categorical programs remained shut off from this source of funds. Furthermore, as the overall level of federal health expenditures climbed, members of Congress looked for ways to check the rise and they found the quickest way to do so was to restrain the growth of the categorical programs. Thus, in one sense, the categorical programs were competing with Medicare and Medicaid for a seemingly limited, although not specifically defined, pool of federal health moneys.

The problems and costs of Medicare were to grow over the years, and grow substantially. In the first year of Medicare, 1966, there were 19 million enrollees and they cost the program $1 billion for medical services. By 1983 there were nearly 30 million enrollees who cost the program $57.4 billion.[26]

The problem was aggravated by a package of social security amendments enacted in 1972 extending Medicare coverage to more people. Persons qualifying for social security disability payments were covered (after a two-year wait) and so was virtually everyone with kidney failure. In 1973, once the legislation expanding the program was in operation, 1.7 million disabled persons joined the Medicare rolls; by 1983 that number had increased to 2.9 million. Kidney patients added 6,400 persons to Medicare's responsibilities in 1973; in 1983 there were 78,000.[27] These groups added significantly to the cost. Medicare costs for the disabled in 1982 were $6.5 billion, of which $2.1 billion was for kidney patients.[28] Thus, the disabled, while only 10 percent of the Medicare population, absorbed 13 percent of the program's expenditures. Kidney patients, only 0.3 percent of that population, absorbed 4 percent.

By the mid-1970s, there was strong pressure to impose constraints, but there was also great difficulty in coming to a consensus as to how to do it. President Ford proposed giving states a fixed amount for Medicaid and considerably more flexibility to run the program. He also proposed putting various restraints on Medicare. Neither idea was accepted by Congress. Herman Talmadge, chairman of the Senate Finance health subcommittee, proposed substantial changes in the two programs designed to eliminate waste and create incentives for efficiency. He suggested a set amount for a specific service regardless of what it cost; if the cost of providing the service was actually less, the hospital could keep the difference. Five years after Ford and Talmadge had proposed these changes, President Reagan was again proposing much the same thing. The difference was that Reagan would have more success.

The Nixon-Congressional Clash

When Richard Nixon became president, the dilemma of the 1980s could be seen on the horizon, but during his first two years in office Nixon offered only modest changes in the statutory design of the health programs originally enacted in the mid-1960s. He proposed moderation, a less rapid expansion of programs and, particularly, holding the line on appropriations. Here he was picking up on an effort started during the Johnson years. Also, he signed into law extensions of the community mental health centers and related programs, legislation expanding and extending various programs to support the training of health care personnel, an extension of the migrant health centers legislation, and creation of a new program to find a solution to cancer, to name a few. It was not until late 1971, in the second half of his first term, that Nixon sought to substantially curtail federal categorical domestic programs. Then he started vetoing legislation to renew and expand these programs, and later impounding funds that had already been appropriated for their operation.

Nixon's impoundment program started somewhat cautiously. The process upon which it was built—congressional directives to the president to, in fact, make selective impoundments—had been started during the Johnson years.

The struggle between the executive and legislature over who should have the final say as to the level of federal spending had been going on virtually since the first days of the Republic. The standard procedure for making funds available to the president was for Congress to write and pass appropriations acts in response to requests by the president. Once funds were enacted, the chief executive had only limited authority not to spend appropriated funds he did not want to spend. He did not have the prerogative of vetoing specific items in appropriations acts that some governors had. Appropriations acts were, of course, the principal device Congress had, beyond the authorizing legislation itself, of spelling out how federal policy should be executed. The appropriation of funds for a particular program meant that program was to continue, in the view of Congress, even if the president disagreed. If the purpose of the program no longer existed—for example, if funds had been appropriated for the purchase of weapons but a war had ended before they were used—the president did not have to spend them.

As the fiscal crunch created by the Vietnam war became more serious during the Johnson years, Congress became increasingly concerned about the level of federal spending. Thus, in the last fiscal year of the Johnson presidency, which started July 1, 1968, Congress directed the president to cut $6 billion from the accumulation of appropriations bills as they had been enacted by Congress. It was left to Nixon to carry through with this obligation when he took office in January 1969. Another, but more limited, grant of impoundment authority was given to Nixon by Congress during his first year in office. In response to both congressional mandates, Nixon impounded more than had been directed by Congress, mostly in the area of public works. At first, health programs were immune to the Nixon device. But the stage was being set for him to act on them, as well.[29]

In January 1970, Nixon vetoed the first version of the fiscal 1970 appropriations bill for the Department of Health, Education and Welfare on the grounds that it exceeded by too much his budget request. Congress upheld the veto. Then, in March, eight months into the fiscal year, Nixon signed a second version, which he found acceptable. Although still appropriating more than he wanted by over a half-billion dollars, the measure contained another one of those provisions, one that Congress had worked out with the White House, requiring the president to cut spending in the bill. He could use his discretion as to where those cuts should be made. Congress again was saying, in effect, "We can't cut back further, but go ahead and impound anyway."

In the meantime, Congress was setting the stage for another device to deal with the increasingly unstable economic situation. It passed in the summer of 1970 the Economic Stabilization Act that gave the president authority to freeze wages and prices, authority Nixon finally used in the summer of 1971, and that was to be used longer and more aggressively in the health sector than in any other sector of the economy.

Then in June 1970 Nixon vetoed the Hill-Burton hospital facility and construction amendments of 1970. The veto was overridden, and that action set the stage for the ensuing impoundment battle in the federal courts. Those lawsuits challenged the Nixon administration's impoundment of funds appropriated for fiscal 1973. The Hill-Burton program had been responsible for the construction of thousands of hospitals throughout the country. By 1970 the program was beginning to become an anachronism in federal health policy (it would be eliminated in 1974) as an excess of beds became one of the causes of rapidly rising hospital costs. Nixon was critical of the measure, in part because it authorized $2.8 billion in grants and loans over three years for the construction and modernization of hospitals; he wanted to eliminate the grant program. But his major objection was a provision mandating that he spend funds appropriated for certain health programs.

The Hill-Burton amendments carried that provision because when Congress was in the final stages of considering the bill, the Senate was having second thoughts about the procedure of giving the president impoundment authority, particularly as it affected health programs, and it decided to include in the Hill-Burton bill a "must spend" provision. It said, in section 601 of the act, that all funds appropriated for Public Health Service programs through fiscal 1973 "shall remain available for obligation and expenditure until such end of the fiscal year."[30]

The report of the House-Senate conference committee, which wrote the final version for the law, said, "The purpose of this amendment is to prevent administratively imposed freezes, reductions, and rollbacks from applying to health programs authorized under these acts."[31] In other words, the president had to spend the funds; he could not impound them under the general authority in the appropriations act to reduce spending. Congress was clearly ambivalent about what it was doing.

In his June 22 veto message, Nixon criticized this provision on the grounds that it would "significantly restrict presidential options in managing federal expenditures."[32] As it turned out, he was correct, for the courts, relying on this provision, ultimately forced Nixon to release health funds he had impounded.

Nixon, although he recognized the threat of the language, ultimately ignored it, and he also kept on vetoing legislation.

In 1972, Nixon ran for reelection. That year was also the first full year of his wage-price freeze, and one in which he did further battle with Congress over the way he was conducting the Vietnam War. Nixon in 1972 also vetoed not one but two health appropriation measures. The first bill was vetoed in August, and the veto was sustained by Congress. The next bill, which contained less money but was still more than a half-billion dollars over the president's request, was pocket-vetoed in October after Congress adjourned for the presidential and congressional elections. This measure, like the 1970 and 1971 bills, contained authority for the president legally to impound funds, but that authority, in Nixon's view, would still not allow him to scale back spending sufficiently. Thus, he vetoed the measure, and another effort, on election eve, to develop new impoundment authority in a third bill collapsed when the Senate dug in its heels. Congress then adjourned and Nixon, of course, went on to win the election by a substantial vote.

When the new Congress convened in 1973, somewhat intimidated by the president's show of strength, its leaders did not attempt to enact a third HEW appropriations bill for fiscal 1973, which by then was more than six months over; instead, HEW was funded for the rest of that fiscal year through a make-shift appropriations bill, a substitute called a continuing resolution, used when regular funding bills were not enacted by the start of the new fiscal year. This bill set the department's spending at the level in the vetoed appropriations bill. No extensive impoundments, as had been permitted previously, were to be allowed under this authority. Although that resolution for fiscal 1973 continued funding for a number of health programs that Nixon wanted to eliminate or substantially phase down, he signed it because it affected more than just HEW, and without it a number of federal agencies would be without funds and would have to shut down. This was the appropriations bill that was in force for health programs when the impoundment cases were argued in the federal courts.

Even though Nixon signed the measure, he did not intend to spend all the funds appropriated, as GOP senators made clear during the final debate on the bill. Instead, Nixon used the spending levels he initially recommended in his budget proposal, and refused to release more funds to the agencies to run their programs. He was now impounding health funds against the explicit wishes of Congress (previously he had impounded other funds, mostly those for public works projects); the battle was joined; and before the 1973 fiscal year ended on June 30, 1973, the president's team was taken to court first by organizations representing highway programs and thereafter by ones representing health programs. They were trying to force him to spend the appropriated funds. The lawsuits with regard to the health programs relied, in part, on the provision in the Hill-Burton act of 1970, as well as on the language of the appropriations act itself. The administration argued against the legality of the 1970 anti-impoundment provision. The courts, however, ruled against the president and directed the administration to spend the funds.

One health program that played a central role in the impoundment debate was the community mental health centers program. Started in the early 1960s, by 1973 it was one of the more ambitious and successful of the categorical grant health programs. In 1970, with Nixon in the White House, the program was given new authority—the duration of the staffing grant was extended, special grants for centers serving poverty areas were created, and programs for providing mental health services to children were started.

When the program was first enacted, its authors believed that when the original staffing grant ran out, state and local governments, the communities that the centers served, and third-party payers, such as insurance companies and Medicare and Medicaid, would provide the funds that heretofore had been provided by the federal grant. Indeed, the grant had been declining in size over that period in anticipation of this. But the outside support was not readily forthcoming. While the committees that had created the program—the House Commerce Committee and the Senate Labor and Public Welfare Committee—had anticipated that Medicare and Medicaid at some point would begin paying for the cost of care delivered to their beneficiaries by the centers program, the two committees that had responsibility for Medicare and Medicaid—Finance in the Senate and Ways and Means in the House—jealously watched over those programs preventing other federal programs from gaining access to their funds.

President Nixon signed the 1970 legislation, but it was to be the last time he supported mental health centers. Within a year he called for their phase-out, and when that call went unheeded by Congress he impounded appropriated funds.

This period for mental health centers, as well as for many other health programs, was a crucial one, and when in the second half of his first term Nixon began to clamp down on domestic spending, the CMHC program was at the center of the storm. All health programs were popular on Capitol Hill, and the CMHC program one of the most popular. It was supported by effective organizations that were tied into larger lobby coalitions. The Executive Branch is generally accepted as the most effective single lobby in Washington, but when others combine in opposition it may be outmatched. Thus it was in the health arena in the early 1970s.

The organizations supporting the CMHC program took on the president when he impounded funds in 1973 and successfully got that decision reversed and the funds, over $52 million, released. The core of the argument against the president was the provision in the 1970 Hill-Burton legislation requiring that appropriated funds be spent. Judge Gerhard Gesell of the U.S. District Court for the District of Columbia found that language decisive, and he also found Congress clearly favored the CMHC program, as he apparently personally did, too:

> The Court concludes that Congress intended to require a full commitment of the fiscal 1973 appropriated funds by the end of the fiscal year. This intent is established by the following facts and circumstances, among others. Through the act, Congress has constructed an elaborate scheme to advance the cause of community mental health treatment, and has continually appropriated money to achieve the purposes of the act. The object of the act is to provide federal money to establish new community mental health centers and programs throughout the nation. . . . In the face of vast unmet mental health needs throughout the nation, Congress has continuously appropriated money for new grants to extend the benefits of the act. The act was never viewed by Congress as a demonstration program to get communities to follow the example of others and start their own centers, but rather a national effort to redress the presently wholly inadequate measures being taken to meet increasing mental health treatment needs.[33]

Gesell consequently in August 1973 directed HEW to promptly complete processing applications for new centers and dispense the funds. It was a major victory not only for the mental health centers program, but also for other health programs, which were to win similar court directives. Now Congress and the Executive Branch were clearly in an adversary relationship. From then on, Congress was much more explicit in writing health legislation.

The CMHC program continued to grow. In 1975, Congress enacted legislation extending and expanding the program and directing quite specifically how it was to be carried out by the Executive Branch. It was one of several reactions by Congress to the Nixon's administration's attempt to eliminate health and other social programs by administrative fiat. In order to ensure that NIMH would administer the program the way Congress wanted, the 1973 act stipulated nine services a mental health center had to provide—this was, if anything, more comprehensive than before.

The CMHC program was not the only one to sue the administration for release of impounded funds. Constituencies for seven health programs, including those who would receive the funds, such as state governments, went to court, all with various degrees of success, to get funds freed. In addition to the centers program, organizations seeking funds impounded for the Hill-Burton hospital construction, regional medical, several training, and alcohol and drug programs successfully protested the administration's actions.

Presidental vetoes of health appropriation measures were, however, only the tip of the iceberg in the struggle between Congress and the Executive Branch over federal spending for health. Nixon's impoundment policy had major long-term ramifications for the way the country's governmental structure works. It led to enactment by Congress in 1974 of the Congressional Budget and Anti-Impoundment Act, which Nixon signed a few weeks before he resigned, and to a substantial increase in the congressional infrastructure. In any institution there is a natural tendency to grow and expand staff and other resources, and Congress has been no exception. Indeed, with each congressional reorganization act, the most recent at this point having been passed in 1970, the infrastructure of Congress had been strengthened. But the great stress between President Nixon and Congress, exemplified first by his impoundment attempts and later by the impeachment effort, dramatically accelerated the movement of Congress toward institutional independence. The 1974 Congressional Budget Act was, in a sense, the climax of that stressful relationship.

That act created three new congressional entities—the Congressional Budget Office and two budget committees, one for the House and another for the Senate. With the additional infrastructure and staff created by this act, Congress would have the capacity to analyze carefully the president's budget and thus make judgments about it and a host of other issues. It also meant that Congress would look at the budget as a whole rather than as a dozen or more pieces as represented by the various appropriation bills, as had been the case until 1974. At the same time, the staff capacity for individual members in both the House and Senate was expanded and committees began to develop larger cadres of professionals who soon would have a full reservoir of knowledge about the programs over which those panels had responsibility.

Never again was Congress to expose itself to such flagrant abuse by a chief executive as Nixon had rendered by his impoundment attempts. Congress from then on would have a bureaucracy as formidable as that of the president, if not as large, and the confrontation between 1600 Pennsylvania Avenue and Capitol Hill would, over the long run, show itself regardless of whether the two were controlled by members of the same political party or by different parties. If Congress was to let the president dominate, as Ronald Reagan dominated during his first year, it would be because the president had the votes to support his policies, and not because he was arbitrarily and unilaterally exercising questionable executive powers.

The impoundment provisions of the 1974 act spelled out in detail the circumstances under which the president could permanently, or even temporarily, impound funds already appropriated by Congress, and gave Congress the opportunity in each case to reject the president's request. Without congressional consent the president could no longer unilaterally withhold funds.

Kennedy and Nixon on NHI

The term "national health insurance" has become a catch-all phrase that means different things to different people, but generically it is a system of health insurance in which the federal government is heavily involved, either because it finances most or all of the health care available under the program, or stipulates what care will or will not be available, at least through that program. National health insurance also generally, but not always, means that everyone has access to most essential health care.

There are several limited national health programs in the United States today in which the federal government is deeply involved, ones that ensure health care for only a limited group of individuals but could serve as the foundation for a larger program providing health insurance for everyone. Medicare is a health insurance program for those 65 years old and over, the disabled and persons with chronic kidney disease. Each of the armed services has a health program in which it provides direct care and insurance for its active-duty members, retirees and their dependents. The Veterans Administration either provides direct care or pays for care primarily for veterans with disabilities resulting from their military service and for poor, aged veterans who are unable to pay for their own care. Many poor people have access to health care through Medicaid.

There are several key issues that always arise in any debate over national health insurance. One is universality, which means that the program should apply to everyone—rich, poor, employed, unemployed—and that each person is guaranteed a certain level of benefits. For some, universality means also that the program applies to everyone in the same way. This can be an important distinction because it means not only that everyone is guaranteed a certain level of health care, but also that everyone has access to the same health care system—the poor person as well as the rich can theoretically get service from the Park Avenue doctor. The two-class (or more) system of health care is particularly bothersome to those who seek a more egalitarian social system in this country.

Other important features are copayments and deductibles—the devices used to make the patient share in the cost of the health care he or she receives. If copayments and deductibles are eliminated, the argument goes, people will seek care when they need it, and get only what they need, and thus stay healthier, so lessening the cost of care in the long run. Copayments and deductibles may deter people from seeking health care immediately, but they also lower the cost of the program.

A third important element in the national health insurance debate is the concept of prospective budgeting, or setting a limit on how much will be spent each year for health care. This can be done in one of several ways, either by establishing an overall limit, a national budget, which, like all budgets, could be divided up according to a set formula, or by set limits on what the national system would pay for a particular element of care—for example, a day in the hospital or a tonsillectomy. Whatever approach might be used meant controlling reimbursements, something that wasn't provided for under the original Medicare-Medicaid legislation. It was the only way, some theorists argued, to control inflation in health care costs, which for decades have been running ahead of inflation in consumer prices generally. And it is this inflation that has scared politicians away from enacting legislation giving the federal government a more substantial role in paying for health care.

All debates over national health insurance in essence became efforts to fill the gaps in existing health insurance coverage so that everyone would, through one device or another, be assured of access to adequate health services, and all debates essentially boiled down, as most public policy debates do, to cost. Some argued that the only way to fill the gaps would be to mandate comprehensive coverage for everyone through a national program run and financed by the federal government. The cost to the federal government, they conceded, would be substantial, but in the long run the nation would be spending less on health care, and moreover the cost issue was irrelevant because in the last analysis it was only a matter of from which pocket—public or private—bills were paid.

But politicians more concerned with the bottom line of the federal budget argued for achieving the same goal without the dollars flowing through the federal Treasury, and as this approach was pursued more gaps opened up; always the first to fall through these gaps were the poor. Thus, the debate over national health insurance, in a larger context, became one that pitted the liberal ethic ("It is the responsibility of government to take care of those who cannot take care of themselves") against the conservative ethic ("If the free enterprise system is allowed to work unfettered by government restraint everyone will be able to adequately care for themselves").

In this debate it would be easy to ensure proper health care for the able-bodied worker and his or her family. The employer could be required to purchase insurance, and since this was a predominantly healthy group the expense was tolerable. Even the unemployed—those seeking jobs but unable to find them—were easy (i.e. relatively inexpensive) to take care of, particularly if they were unemployed for only short periods—their former employers could be required to continue health insurance coverage for a year or so. Those who had long-term illnesses could be fairly easily covered by a back-up federal health insurance program, or catastrophic coverage, that would take effect after a person had spent a particular amount of his or her own money—say $3,000—on the illness.

As the national health insurance debates flowed and ebbed over the years, consensus would be reached on how to finance comprehensive health care for virtually everyone except for the poor and near-poor—that became the gap impossible to close, and the reason was the cost to the federal Treasury. It was, in essence, a matter of upgrading the Medicaid program that paid for health care services for some, but not all, of the poor.

When the term "national health insurance" first emerged in the early decades of this century it meant a program mandated by the federal government but financed and run by the states. Later, during the New Deal, it came to mean a program, like social security, that would be largely or totally financed by the federal government but in which there would be little additional federal involvement; it was to be only a mechanism for financing health care.

A few years after the creation of Medicare in 1965, efforts to enact national health insurance again emerged, this time under the sponsorship of Edward Kennedy and organized labor, primarily the United Auto Workers. Richard Nixon, two years into his presidency, also offered a national health insurance plan, and the congressional hoppers were becoming filled with health insurance proposals of one sort or another. But it was the Kennedy and Nixon plans in their various forms that provided the anchors for the NHI debate that was to continue through the Carter administration.

In the Kennedy-UAW lexicon, national health insurance meant a program financed by the federal government with funds gathered through a payroll tax that would pay for all necessary health care for everyone. No one would have to pay any part of the health care bill—either a deductible at the beginning of service, say the cost of the first day of hospital care (which is what Medicare beneficiaries must pay) or a copayment such as 20 percent of the physician's bill (which is also what Medicare beneficiaries must pay). Under the Kennedy-labor plan, which became known as the Health Security Act, a commission each year would establish a national health budget and each region of the country would get its proportionate share. Each hospital would be given a set amount for treating everyone who came through its doors that year, and its budget would be determined by its costs in the previous year, plus an additional amount to compensate for inflation and help it to buy new equipment and otherwise improve services. Limits would be set on what doctors could charge for a specific service. This budgeting device provided a mechanism for controlling inflation in health care costs, an increasingly worrisome phenomenon for federal health policy-makers.

The traditional role of insurance companies would have been eliminated under the Health Security Act, since they would no longer be underwriting health insurance policies; that meant that they would not be making a profit (or suffering a loss) on the gamble they took by selling health insurance. If insurance companies were to have any role under the Kennedy-labor national health insurance program it would simply be to pay bills in behalf of the government, or to serve the government as an intermediary as under Medicare.

The Health Security Act after it was first introduced in 1971 became the standard for the all-inclusive government-run health insurance program, and for many it came to mean socialized medicine. It was not socialized medicine, however; but the description became an easy, and clearly pejorative, one to use and helped to polarize the debate. It was not socialized medicine because health care providers, primarily doctors and hospitals, did not become part of the federal apparatus. They would continue to work in the same way—individual or group practices for doctors and nonprofit or for-profit corporations for hospitals.

Nixon's bill, the National Health Insurance Partnership Act, consisted of two parts—the Family Health Insurance Plan and the National Health Insurance Standards Act. The former was a federally financed plan to provide health insurance for all low-income families, thus, in effect, expanding the Medicaid mandate. The second, financed largely by private funds, set standards for employer health insurance programs and required coverage of employees. But this plan could not win the support needed because, under it, too many people—approximately 40 million—still would lack coverage, the benefit package was severely limited, and it basically built upon the existing system without providing any significant changes designed to make it more efficient. The plan was to be withdrawn at the end of Nixon's first term.

Nixon's plan attempted to combine the principles of the liberal Democratic ethic of a guaranteed right to health care with features ensuring that its cost could more easily be controlled than Medicare's had been. The Kennedy plan, in contrast, picked up where Harry Truman's national health insurance plan left off by proposing guaranteed health insurance coverage for everyone, covering virtually all health care costs and paid for through a special payroll tax.

Outlining his health insurance plan, Nixon, in his health message to Congress on February 18, 1971, initially stressed not the need for adequate health care for everyone, but instead the rising cost of health care, which had climbed 170 percent since 1960, with much of the additional expenditures coming from the federal Treasury. "What are we getting for all this money?" he asked rhetorically. Answering his own question, he said that 60 percent of the growth in health care expenditures had gone not for newer and better care, but instead for higher prices for the same care. There were other shortcomings, Nixon said: inadequate distribution of personnel and resources, and too little prevention, resulting in an excess of intensive care. In short, he argued, "Costs have skyrocketed but values have not kept pace. We are investing more of our nation's resources in the health of our people but we are not getting a full return on our investment." Good health care, he went on, "should be readily available to all of our citizens."[34]

But Nixon was not interested simply in starting up a national health insurance program. He said he wanted to develop a new national health strategy, one that would assure equal access to health care, balance the supply of health care resources with the demand, organize the health care system more efficiently, and build on existing strengths. Key elements in his reorganization plan were to provide federal support for the creation of health maintenance organizations—a proposal from which he later backed away—improve methods for financing medical education, and provide better programs to prevent disease and poor health.

If Nixon saw the need for a national health insurance plan to help cut costs and stabilize the nation's health care system, he was also interested in getting reelected in 1972, and he saw Ted Kennedy, whose popularity was then rising, pushing his own plan. NHI was now an issue that could not be ignored in presidential politics.

Kennedy in August 1970 had introduced his first version of national health insurance legislation backed by the United Auto Workers, and about the same time a similar proposal backed by the AFL-CIO had been introduced in the House by Representative Martha Griffiths, a Democrat from Michigan. In 1971 the two combined and revised their bills, offering a joint package, to be called the Health Security Act. This became the standard Kennedy national health insurance bill.

The genesis for the Kennedy bill, however, dates back to shortly after the enactment of the Medicare and Medicaid programs in 1965. That effort had been long fought, as we have seen, but for some it was only one step along the way to a full-fledged national health insurance program. Walter Reuther, then head of the United Auto Workers, was a proponent, and after the programs were underway he set the stage for the next effort.

Reuther's first step was to hire Max Fine as one of his aides. Fine had worked in HEW since the advent of the Kennedy administration primarily helping to create the political climate necessary to win enactment of Medicare. The two set to work putting together the technical expertise necessary for writing a national health insurance bill and for developing the grass-roots support that would be necessary to make the new effort a prominent legislative undertaking. Quickly, within a year or so, the costs of Medicare were causing problems and it became clear that the next stage would have to provide more than simply a mechanism for financing health care. It would have to make some changes in the way health care was financed—namely through an open-ended reimbursement system that relied on payments from a third party, an insurance company, rather than the patient.

Reuther, Fine and Melvin Glasser, who throughout this period was in charge of UAW's social programs, put together a technical committee to write the new plan. Once Republicans took over the White House in 1969 and it was clear a new Democratic president would not be able to offer the NHI proposal, they created the Committee for National

Health Insurance to take over both the drafting and lobbying activities. Fine became its executive director.

Reuther and Fine went to Kennedy early in 1969 to persuade him to take on their NHI cause. They chose Kennedy because he had already expressed an interest in health issues, but also because he clearly was a presidential prospect, having taken over the political mantle of the Kennedy family following the murder of his brother Robert in 1968. For NHI to become successful it needed to have the whole-hearted support of the president.[35] Kennedy in 1969 was a member of the Senate Labor and Public Welfare health subcommittee, which made NHI a natural interest for him. Two years later the opportunity to exploit that interest would be expanded when Ralph Yarborough, then the subcommittee chairman, lost his reelection bid and Kennedy was able to take over the panel.

While that subcommittee was not the primary one for considering national health insurance legislation, any such bills would be jointly referred to it, as well as to the Finance Committee, which did have primary responsibility, and it would give Kennedy considerable visibility in the health arena.

Several things happened to dim this plan, however. In June 1969, within six months of the time Reuther and Fine had persuaded him to take on the national health insurance effort, Kennedy, through negligent driving, caused the death of a young woman at Chappaquidick on Martha's Vineyard. This incident thwarted Kennedy's presidential ambitions in the near future and perhaps permanently, thus blocking the path to the White House for the UAW's national health insurance plan.

Then Reuther, who was the originating and prime force behind the plan, was killed in an airplane crash in May 1970, and with his death a good deal of creativeness went out of the NHI effort. While Reuther's successors, first Leonard Woodcock and later Douglas Fraser, were committed to national health insurance, neither had Reuther's driving desire to push through its enactment.

Kennedy, when he took on the leadership of the national health insurance effort for the Democrats, understood that to be successful he would have to work through a coalition, and an ever-expanding one. Thus, he immediately pushed to have his 1970 bill consolidated with legislation developed by the AFL-CIO and sponsored in the House by Martha Griffiths. But beyond that, he knew he would have to work closely with committee leaders—Wilbur Mills in the House and Russell Long in the Senate—and with the president.[36]

Although the cost issue was a strong motivation when Kennedy introduced the consolidated version of the Health Security Act on January 25, 1971, it was not his primary motive for sponsoring the bill, as it had been for Nixon. Instead, he used the proposal as a vehicle to further articulate the liberal Democratic dogma that later was to become the test for Democratic presidential candidates. "I believe that in America today, health care is a right for all, not just a privilege for the few," he said, as he began his remarks.[37] The health care system in the United States was so warped, he argued, that in order to insure adequate health care for everyone, the financing of health care had to be redesigned and the task taken away from the insurance industry, which had bungled the job. The key to the new financing mechanism would be a prospective budget to cover the cost of health care for the entire nation; it would be divided among sections of the country according to estimated need. Hospitals would be given their own budgets, and would be expected to live within them. Not only would health care be a right of citizenship, but the federal government would be the only mechanism capable of doing the job.

Kennedy took on the medical profession as well. The task of changing the present system would be tough, Kennedy said. "Throughout our society today, there is perhaps no institution more resistant to change than the organized medical profession."[38]

The "private health insurance industry has failed us," he went on. "It fails to control costs. It fails to control quality. It provides partial benefits, not comprehensive benefits; acute care, not preventive care. It ignores the poor and the medically indigent." Because private insurance usually paid only for the cost of hospital care, the health insurance industry forced doctors and patients to "resort to wasteful and inefficient use of hospital facilities, thereby giving further impetus to the already soaring cost of hospital care and unnecessary strains on health manpower."[39]

Now the health care industry had become a giant that must be slain by the public servant. It was admittedly a huge industry, accounting in 1971 for 7.7 percent of the gross national product while spending a total of $83.3 billion. In 1950, the nation had spent only $12.7 billion, or 4.4 percent of GNP, on health care. In 1960, national health care expenditures had been only $26.9 billion, or 5.3 percent of GNP. In 1967, a year after Medicare and Medicaid had begun operation, expenditures were $51.3 billion, or 6.4 percent of GNP. The industry continued to grow, and in 1981 expenditures were $286.6 billion, or 9.8 percent of GNP.[40] Both Kennedy and Nixon were trying to tame the monster.

Kennedy saw his initial commitment with national health insurance not so much a dedication to a particular bill or concept as an opportunity to take hold of a major domestic issue and pursue it, massage it, and gain the public's attention and interest. He saw the legislation as a vehicle, and he used that vehicle throughout the early 1970s to hold hearings and stimulate interest in the concept of national health insurance. He was largely successful in doing this, and his success was in large part due to his characterization of the health care and insurance industries as the villains. It gave the knight in shining armor something to shoot at.

Responding to Kennedy, Nixon attempted to stay friendly with both the medical care industry and the insurance industry. In order to accomplish his health goals, Nixon said, it was not necessary to nationalize the nation's health industry, and there was "no need to eliminate an entire segment of our private economy and at the same time add a multibillion dollar responsibility to the federal budget. Such a step should not be taken unless all other steps failed. More than that, such action would be dangerous. It would deny people the right to choose how they would pay for their health care. It would remove competition from the insurance system, and with it an incentive to experiment and innovate." Under a nationalized system of health care, Nixon said, no one—consumer, practitioner, institution—would have any incentive to hold down costs, and thus the "only way that utilization could be effectively regulated and costs effectively restrained . . . would be if the federal government made a forceful, tenacious effort to do so." Federal personnel under the Kennedy plan would have to approve the budgets of local hospitals, set fee schedules for local doctors, and take "other steps which could easily lead to the complete federal domination of all American medicine."[41] Nixon implied that Kennedy's scheme would be socialized medicine, thus politicizing the issue, just as Robert Taft had done two decades earlier.

Kennedy and Nixon differed on the causes of rising health care costs. In testimony before the Finance Committee that spring, Kennedy placed the responsibility squarely on the health insurance industry, and argued that on its record it deserved to be put out of business. "Only the health insurance industry stands to lose if the health security act is passed—and that industry has shown it has neither the ability nor the will to control costs or promote efficiency." Although his program would be costly—about $60 billion in its first year—Kennedy maintained there would be no new money involved, for $60 billion was what the nation would spend on health care that year anyway under the present system.[42]

This was, he argued, the major distinction between his proposal and the administration's. The Nixon bill, he testified, would "place an even greater responsibility in the hands of the industry and increase the amount of funds handled by the industry—a windfall worth billions of dollars a year for the private carriers."[43]

As the 92d Congress began in 1971, it looked like a national health insurance program might be enacted, for there was substantial support for "doing something" in Congress and the presidency was strongly pushing a measure that it hoped would gain the support of a broad constituency. But that expectation was quickly shattered. As he began the second half of his first term, Nixon took a different leadership tack. He became much more belligerent in his approach to Congress and in his efforts to hold down federal spending, as he had been earlier in his impoundments. Inflation generally was becoming a problem. Health care prices by 1970 were rising by 7.3 percent a year, while prices generally in the economy were rising by only 4.3 percent. By the summer of 1971 Nixon had imposed a 90-day wage and price freeze and then instituted a program to control inflation in the health care sector that would last until the spring of 1974. When the 92d Congress adjourned in the fall of 1972, it was in a contentious mood. The country was moving into another presidential election, this time involving an incumbent president who, although the full dimensions were yet to be revealed, was already clearly tainted with unsavory behavior. It was not the time to institute a national health insurance program.

The Rise and Fall of HMOs and Training Programs

Among the many contradictions in Nixon's presidency, a major one was the way he approached health issues in the early years of his incumbency. One manifestation of that contradiction was his initial strong embrace of a new federal program to promote the development of health maintenance organizations, an ardor that ultimately cooled. In the process, though, the stage was set for creation of still another major federal health initiative, and behind the impetus was the increasingly strong desire to do something about rising health care costs.

The legislation creating the health maintenance organization program anticipated that HMOs would start opening up all over the country soon after its enactment, rather than developing in increments over the years. It was also expected to quickly have a significant impact on the way health care was delivered. An HMO would provide comprehensive general health care in a unified setting at a predetermined cost. It was to be a substantial improvement over existing ways of delivering health care. For those who used an HMO it would be equivalent to national health insurance.

Although not always called such, health maintenance organizations had been around for fifty years. Conceptually, from the point of view of a sound health care delivery system, the HMO was very attractive. It was usually a single building or a collection of buildings located nearby one another. If the inpatient service or hospital was not part of the core organization, it was, nevertheless, usually easily accessible. The HMO provided a full array of health care services, and thus practitioners, to its members through a single administrative unit; in health care lingo it was called an organized setting.

A patient's needs, whatever they were, could, except in the most extreme cases, be taken care of through this one program. Furthermore, the emphasis was on preventive care and outpatient treatment, thus lessening the need for hospitalization, the most expensive element in health care. If unusual care was called for, such as a heart transplant, the HMO had contracted with a qualified facility that could do the operation.

Not anyone could walk into an HMO and receive treatment; one had to be a member, and becoming one involved application and acceptance, much as one became a member of an insurance plan. In a practical sense, an HMO was an insurance plan that provided its own care, and this had caused much of the controversy.

Rather than paying for each service after it was rendered, an HMO member paid a set amount in advance on a monthly or yearly basis to cover all the care he or she might need during the period. Thus, by emphasizing prevention, the HMO was betting that it could make money on the patient because the patient would not need costly services. The HMO, just as the typical health insurance company, was, in the parlance of economists, at risk.

The HMO approach to health care had always been controversial. When the first plans, then called prepaid health plans, were started in the early 1930s, doctors opposed them, and it was finally that opposition four decades later that cooled the Nixon administration to the idea. For whatever reasons—the threat of competition or the genuine professional belief that the prepaid plan would result in inferior care—organized medicine, although not all doctors, opposed HMOs and particularly federal support for them.

In 1932, for example, the *Journal of the American Medical Association* warned that prepaid practice meant "solicitation of patients, destructive competition among professional groups, inferior medical service, loss of personal relationship of patient and physician and demoralization of the profession."[44] Since the plan was a financing as well as a health care delivery scheme, in many states the insurance commissioners and legislatures were persuaded that HMOs were really insurance companies in addition to whatever else they might be, and therefore should be regulated under state insurance laws. Often on these grounds, HMOs were prevented from doing business.

By the 1980s, the medical profession had backed off from that criticism and largely accepted the HMO as an integral part of the nation's health care delivery system. Also, by then states had for the most part had enacted legislation to permit HMOs to operate without encumbrance.

The HMO became particularly attractive to those who believed that the federal government was so heavily involved in the nation's health care system, either through the purchase of care or through regulation, that there was no longer competition in the health market. They viewed the HMO as the principal device by which the traditional competition of the marketplace could be reintroduced to the delivery of health care services. It offered an alternative to the usual way of getting health care, and since health care received through an HMO was usually less expensive, in the aggregate, than fee-for-service care, the HMO would be competitive in both style and cost.

Nevertheless, there were serious and legitimate concerns about the HMO concept, both in its ability to provide care to a substantial segment of the population and in the possibility that individual HMOs under financial stress would skimp on care needed by their members. Although data clearly showed that HMOs used substantially less hospital care than traditional fee-for-service health care, HMOs, some thought, might skimp on services when the patient required an unusual amount of care.

HMOs received virtually no support or encouragement from the federal government until the early 1970s, when they caught the fancy of the Nixon administration health policy-makers, precisely because Nixon officials believed HMOs would hold down the rise in health care costs.

Having campaigned on a platform of fiscal austerity and the need for reducing federal expenditures, Nixon sought suggestions from his advisors and got a possible solution to the problem of rising health care costs. Ironically, it was one that required starting a new federal program, a strategy generally denounced by the Nixon administration.

In July 1969, Nixon set the stage for his yet-to-be-developed HMO program. At a press conference called to discuss an HEW report that identified the principal culprit in the health care system as mounting inflation, he said, "We face a massive crisis in [health]. . . . A breakdown in our medical care system. . . ."[45] Nixon said he would not take the easy way out, that proposed by the Democrats, by creating a national health insurance program that would federalize the nation's health care system, but instead would offer creative solutions and improve the cost effectiveness of existing programs.

At that point he did not identify what the solutions might be, HMOs or anything else, but he did plan later to make a major health policy statement and he established a work group to prepare for this.

One of the ideas pursued by this group was the possibility of federal support for HMOs. Paul Elwood, a physician and health policy analyst from Minnesota, had for years been attracted to the benefits of prepaid health plans, because his research showed him that those who used HMOs also used less hospital care; it was a way, he saw, of getting at the problem of rising health care costs. Elwood had attempted to push his idea with the Johnson administration health policy-makers, but they had not been attracted to it. Now he saw the chance to bring his proposals to health policy-makers in the Nixon administration, and they adopted the idea. The first step, HEW officials decided, would be to make it possible for Medicare beneficiaries to select an HMO as the place they would receive treatment. By having Medicare beneficiaries use HMOs, which are paid a lump sum for each person enrolled in the program, Medicare costs could be controlled. The Nixon administration adopted the idea, and in the spring of 1970 as the House Ways and Means Committee was writing amendments to the Medicare and Medicaid programs, the Department of Health, Education and Welfare proposed, and the committee accepted, an amendment that would encourage beneficiaries to use HMOs. That 1970 legislation was never enacted, however.

Then, in June 1970, Elliot Richardson became secretary of HEW and took a keen interest in health policy generally and HMOs in particular.

By the end of the year, Richardson had decided to push for a substantial federal investment in HMOs.

Finally, on February 18, 1971, Nixon sent his first health message to Congress. Its principal focus was his health insurance program, mentioned earlier, but he also proposed enactment of legislation authorizing federal grants to help HMOs get started. Although he acknowledged that care provided by HMOs was good, the quality of care was not his primary reason for proposing a new program. In an HMO, Nixon said, "cost consciousness is fostered. Such an organization cannot afford to waste resources—that costs more money in the short run. But neither can it afford to economize in ways that hurt patients—for that increases long-run expenses."[46]

The message did not spell out the full scope of Nixon's HMO proposal, nor did it describe the full range of the administration's ambitions for the new health care delivery mechanism. Those would be defined in a May departmental white paper on health, and they would be very large. By 1976, 40 million people would be enrolled in 1,700 HMOs, the paper said, if Congress adopted the administration's plan and it was promptly implemented. By 1980, 90 percent of the population could be enrolled in health maintenance organizations.[47]

It was an ambitious proposal, way beyond the realm of possibility even for the most optimistic supporters. Whether that network of HMOs would be needed to provide the substantial relief for Medicare and Medicaid programs the administration was looking for was problematic; the chance of making such a shift was extremely unlikely. But apparently the Nixon administration believed that without that number of people enrolled in HMOs it would not be possible to get enough Medicare beneficiaries into prepaid plans where the costs were predetermined and thus could be controlled.

The only significant obstacle in the Democratically controlled Congress to the HMO proposal at that time was in the Senate Finance Committee, which had jurisdiction over HMOs only as they might relate to the Medicare and Medicaid programs. It was in large part the opposition of the Finance Committee that created the momentum for Congress to enact a new categorical grant program to fund HMOs. In 1971 the committee raised the question of whether the prepayment approach to health care services was likely to result in less than the necessary care required by an individual simply in order to enhance the HMOs' financial situation. If fee-for-service medicine, the panel asked in a September 1971 report, has an "inherent potential for overutilization to maximize profit, does the prepayment approach have an inherent potential for under-servicing to maximize return?"[48]

There were two serious potential concerns about opening up Medicare and Medicaid to HMOs, the Finance Committee argued: the quality of care that might be provided beneficiaries and the possibility of financial windfalls to HMOs. As for the first concern, the committee admitted that most HMOs provided care of a high professional quality, but, it said in a report, "if the government begins on a widespread basis to pay a set sum in advance to an organization in return for the delivery of all necessary care to a group of people, there must be effective means of assuring that such organizations will not be tempted to cut corners on the quality of their care (e.g. by using marginal facilities or by not providing necessary care and services) in order to maximize their return or 'profit.' Under present reimbursement arrangements, although there may be no incentive for efficiency, neither is there an incentive to profit through underservicing and other corner-cutting."[49]

With regard to the second problem, the report went on, "If an HMO were to enroll relatively good risks (i.e. the younger and healthier Medicare beneficiaries), payment to that organization in relation to average per capita non-HMO costs—without accurate actuarial adjustments—could result in 'large windfalls' for the HMO, as the current costs of caring for these beneficiaries might turn out to be much less than Medicare's average per capita costs."[50]

If the Senate Finance Committee was skeptical about the advantages of HMOs, other congressional committees were not. When in 1972 legislation was drafted by the Senate Labor and Public Welfare health subcommittee, that panel argued there was "substantial evidence that HMO enrollees receive high quality care at significantly lower cost—as much as one-fourth to one-third lower than traditional care in some parts of the country."[51] Obviously, then, these plans, once widely enough available, would reap substantial economic benefits for anyone who chose to use them, the committee report suggested. In 1972, Edward Kennedy was in his second year as chairman of the panel and was searching for ways to build the foundation for national health insurance.

Kennedy in those days was approaching health care issues systematically. How did the legislation complement his national health insurance effort? How did it deal with the major problems of quality, cost, maldistribution (of both people and resources), of prevention, of improving our knowledge of biomedical problems? The HMO could make a major contribution to solving these problems—it could improve quality and access; preventive health care could take precedence over cures; and it could help to hold down costs. He made sure the arguments were clearly articulated and there for the record.

Kennedy's panel in its report argued that the fixed-price structure provided a "strong financial incentive" for physicians and hospitals to place "greater emphasis on preventive services to avoid the need for costly, intensive care that can reduce their income." Waste and inefficiency, it said, would not be passed on to the consumer or third-party payers, and because the HMO made a full spectrum of services available through a single organization it was more convenient for the patient.[52]

Despite whatever other advantages might be derived from a vast nationwide network of HMOs, Congress, from the first days the proposal came before it, clearly viewed the scheme as a way of cutting back on the escalation of health care costs. The 1972 report on the new HMO program by Kennedy's committee dwelt on this issue, pointing out that in the decade ending in 1971 the nation's health care expenditures had risen by nearly 200 percent to $75 billion and that a "large portion of that increase went to meet the continuing inflation in health care prices and to subsidize inefficiency and waste in the delivery of health care services."[53] When Congress adjourned in the fall of 1972, however, it had not enacted an HMO program. Thus, when the new Congress convened the next year, the process for HMOs started again from the beginning.

The HMO was also viewed as a way of dealing with some fundamental problems in the nation's health care delivery system—that certain groups of people were not getting adequate health care. When Kennedy's panel filed a second report on the HMO legislation in 1973, it said it this way:

> The committee is deeply concerned over the increasing difficulty scores of millions of Americans continue to experience in obtaining prompt, appropriate health services. . . . While each year more and more dollars are being spent on health care, patients are getting less and less for each dollar spent. We see a health care industry trying to meet 20th century problems with inefficient medical practices and models developed in the 19th century.[54]

This report reflected Kennedy's frustration, one increasingly felt by many in Congress at that time, about the medical care system, and about doctors. It criticized the tendency of physicians to specialize and the scarcity of primary-care physicians. It noted that millions of Americans, not just those living in remote urban and rural areas, were not getting the care they deserved. Thus, it argued, the HMO, because it was more efficient, was "strategic to any attempt to restructure the present practices of delivering health care, and that the federal government must play a lead role in assisting in the development of such organizations."[55]

Until "serious and dramatic attention is given to the role of the federal dollar in reforming the nation's health care delivery capability and efficiency," the Kennedy report continued, Congress can look forward to a "bleaker future in financing" health care.[56] The way to gain leverage from the federal dollar, it said, was by developing a vast network of health maintenance organizations financed largely by the federal government.

If the foundation was being laid for national health insurance, it was also being laid for exceedingly high expectations for the HMO program. HMOs were to be the panacea for all the ills of the nation's health care system. This was an expectation that would be impossible to realize.

As signed into law by President Nixon on December 29, 1973, nearly three years after he first sent his proposal to Capitol Hill, the Health Maintenance Organization Act was much more modest than originally conceived. Both Nixon's 1971 proposal and the bill passed by the Senate in 1972 were substantial, far-reaching measures. The first Senate bill, for example, authorized $5.2 billion over three years for starting up new HMOs and for related efforts. The version signed into law authorized $375 million over three years for projects that were to be more limited in scope.

A lot happened in the intervening years. By the end of 1972, although he had won a substantial victory in that fall's elections, Nixon's incumbency was becoming increasingly tarnished with the Watergate scandal and the tension between Capitol Hill and the White House was escalating. Furthermore, the administration's ardor for HMOs had cooled, in large part in response to the arguments by the American Medical Association that maintained that the proposal provided federal support for a particular kind of medical practice while ignoring others. The price tag of the Senate's 1972 bill, which had been enthusiastically supported by Edward Kennedy, was pared to $1.5 billion by the Senate panel before sending it to the floor, where it was further shaved to $805 million by Kennedy in order to ward off substantial opposition.

In the House, Paul Rogers, the chairman of the House Commerce health subcommittee during this period, had grown very skeptical of the administration's ability to successfully implement health programs without strong congressional guidance. Congress generally and Rogers particularly were becoming increasingly insistent that authorizing legislation detail the specifics of how the program should be run. Rogers did not like the administration's desire for carte blanche on how to administer the HMO program.

But if this were so, Congress increasingly was also moving away from the belief that large grant programs were realistic devices to impose on the nation's health care system. Rogers always had been more fiscally conservative than Kennedy, and now, in an era of rising inflation, wage and price controls and mounting political instability, his conservatism would prevail; Congress was not as willing to authorize large grant programs, and those authorized would be funded more modestly.

Rogers's subcommittee wanted an even more modest bill then sought by the Senate panel. The final measure was much closer to the House version in cost—$375 million in the final bill as opposed to $240 million in the version passed by the House—and it was also more modest in scope.

As signed into law, the measure required that in order to become a federally sanctioned HMO, and thus to be eligible for federal financial support, a program must offer its enrollees eight basic services, ranging from inpatient, outpatient and emergency services to home health services. For an additional fee the HMO could provide a package of supplemental services ranging from nursing, eye and dental care to rehabilitation therapy.

The cost of participating in the program was to be the same for everyone, regardless of medical history, a 30-day annual open-enrollment period was mandated, and the program had to continue providing care to enrollees regardless of the medical care they might need. The measure also overrode state laws that made it difficult for HMOs to organize and required most employers to offer an HMO plan to its employees along with other insurance.

But even if the 1973 HMO law was more modest financially than originally conceived, it nevertheless carried high expectations for HMOs and burdened them with many requirements. It was also very fragile. From the first, as was the case with most federal grant programs, particularly those carrying high expectations, the HMO program was not given the financial support its original architects and constituency anticipated. It had also been the victim of ambivalent feelings on the part of the Nixon administration and of confusing signals from Congress that initially saddled the program with a set of standards it was later to retract as too burdensome.

The problems for the program quickly became apparent as the administration sought to implement the 1973 act and when Congress, later, reviewed it prior to extending it.

When the HMO act came before Congress in 1975, as consideration to renew the program began, congressional health leaders complained about the slowness with which the Nixon and Ford administrations launched it. Only five HMOs had qualified for federal support and only 157 organizations had gotten some kind of exploratory grant.

But Congress also found that the original 1973 act asked too much of HMOs. The "actual requirements of the original act are excessively strict and have the effect of placing developing HMOs at a competitive disadvantage with respect to other parts of the health care system," the 1975 report of the House Commerce Committee said.[57]

Legislation enacted in 1976 extending the program eased some of the more stringent provisions of the early program, but not without opposition. When Congress looked anew at the program it expressed particular concern about the provision that required federally supported HMOs to allow anyone who chose to enroll. This provision, the legislators now found, forced HMOs to take members with heavy health needs, people who would have been rejected by traditional insurance companies. This made it difficult, if not impossible, for all HMOs to compete successfully, in a financial sense, with standard insurance programs.

The 1976 amendments, which extended the HMO program through 1979, scaled back several requirements in the existing law, as had been requested by HMOs themselves and by the Ford administration. The number of services that an HMO was required to provide was pared, and the open enrollment provision was eliminated, except for large and well-established programs.

By 1978, when the HMO program was again to be considered by Congress, the Carter administration was eager to reelevate the program to its original place of glory. Carter saw, just as Nixon had, in HMOs the potential for holding down inflation in health costs. But Carter's HEW was also very critical of the way the previous administration had handled the program.

Hale Champion, Carter's HEW undersecretary, testified before the Senate Labor and Public Welfare health subcommittee in 1978:

> Despite the promises of President Nixon in the early 1970s that by 1976 there would be 1800 prepaid health plans with 40 million enrollees, when we arrived there were only 6.5 million people in 165 HMOs. We found a program that had been systematically undercut . . . was poorly organized, under and inappropriately staffed, and chronically slow in issuing regulations and processing qualified applications. This incompetence had dampened significantly enthusiasm for the HMO concept.[58]

The Carter administration's support of HMOs never faltered. In 1979, Carter's HEW outlined a ten-year strategy to stimulate the growth of HMOs that was nearly as ambitious as that originally pushed by Nixon. If 440 programs were begun by 1990, HEW anticipated that total HMO enrollment in the country would grow from 7.4 million to 19.1 million over the decade, with a cumulative savings during that period of $20 billion. The core of the new plan was an effort by HEW to target its resources at those communities where the payoffs would be the greatest.[59]

It was an expansion of the program that would never occur. The Reagan administration health policy-makers, claiming that the HMO program as a federal effort had achieved success, argued that it no longer deserved federal support. Thus, with the concurrence of Congress, it began withdrawing federal financial backing.

While the HMO program was getting off to a rocky start in the Nixon administration, the federal health policy apparatus was having to come to terms with support for training physicians and other health care practitioners.

Predictions of doctor shortages first started appearing in the 1950s. A 1959 report predicted that the number of doctors trained would have to be increased substantially in order to ensure against a decline in the number of physicians in relation to the population.[60]

In 1971, when it was again time to renew the basic statutory legislation authorizing these programs, Congress was again confronted with data showing continuing shortages; it responded by enacting legislation expanding the program. This new law obligated the federal government to pay medical schools a lump sum for each enrolled student and provide a broader range of support for students, including scholarships and a variety of loans, some of which could later be forgiven if the graduate practiced in shortage areas.

As in previous years, when new training programs were written or existing ones reauthorized, Congress and the administration in 1971 raised the ante for federal support. To qualify for federal grants, schools had to expand enrollment, maintain existing levels of nonfederal support, conduct certain programs such as cooperative interdisciplinary training, and finance, at least in part, the education of poor students. The federal government would have a stronger say in how its dollars would be used.

But the apparent harmony between the administration and Congress over federal support for training was over.

Scarcely was the 1971 law enacted when doubts were raised about the need to train the number of physicians envisioned by the authors of that legislation, and the Nixon administration in 1973 began publicly voicing concern about the prospects of a doctor surplus. Besides, the program was costing nearly $100 million a year, and the administration was committed to cutting back on federal expenditures. Here was a program whose elimination could be easily justified. Even Kennedy, who had seen training programs as another way of building the base for national health insurance by making physicians more widely available throughout the country and by focusing federal support to promote the training of more general practitioners, would have an increasingly hard time justifying the program.

By 1974 medical schools had increased enrollment substantially and had become more stable financially. There was no longer the need to increase the aggregate supply of health care personnel. Now the problems were exclusively ones of geographic and specialty distribution.

The administration argued against using federal grants to medical schools to solve the distribution problem. It wanted to terminate the program. Congress extended the program in 1976, but with increasing concern over the federal investment in health in all areas, support for training health care personnel was clearly on the downward slide.

Federal support by this time had become untenable as a matter of public policy, for it was a matter of gross inequity. Federal dollars were being used to subsidize the professional education of people who would, within a few years after graduation, be among the very top income earners in the country. They could thus be asked to borrow the money for their training, even if they had to pay it back at high interest rates.

By 1980, when legislation supporting health training efforts was again considered by Congress, the total number of physicians, in the view of most experts, was clearly sufficient to meet the nation's needs. Indeed, there was likely to be a surplus within a decade. But by 1980, federal support for medical schools and students had become such a solid fixture that the schools argued it would be unfair to drop it, for to do so would create instability and force them to substantially raise tuition, which in some cases was already as high as $13,000 per year. However, Congress did drop support and medical schools were able to go it alone.

The centerpiece of the nation's medical training apparatus is the medical center, which groups medical schools, hospitals and research facilities together. This is a highly complex and sophisticated collection. The centers grew out of biomedical research facilities, and federal support for them was the precursor of federal support for training per se.

The nation's most renowned physicians—doctors who are not only highly skilled but highly specialized—are associated with medical centers. It is at the centers that they build not only their reputations, but the complicated infrastructure and support system for carrying out their research and practice. Students associated with these centers naturally seek to emulate their leaders—in prestige, in specialized skill and in wealth. When these young doctors begin their independent careers, they naturally, in most cases, seek out arrangements that will do for them what they have just seen done for their teachers.

Thus, by the mid-1970s there was not only a surplus of physician specialists and a paucity of generalists practicing primary care, but the specialists lived and worked in areas near the medical centers.

This was despite the fact that the actual number of physicians and the number of physicians in relation to the population had grown steadily since 1940. In 1965 there were 145.5 physicians per 100,000 people. By 1970, a few years after enactment of federal legislation to encourage training of more doctors, the ratio had climbed to 154.5. By 1975, when, it is now generally accepted, supply and need came in balance, there were 377,350 physicians, and a ratio of 173.1 per 100,000 people. Projections showed that by 1990 there would be nearly 600,000 physicians, which would increase the ratio to 245.[61] Still, more doctors were needed who would practice primary-care medicine and practice it in the less-attractive parts of the country.

The role of the primary-care physicians is to be the first contact with the patient. While the primary-care doctor may refer the patient to a specialist for further treatment, he can take care of about 90 percent of the health needs of the country. Also, the primary-care physician usually charges less than the specialist, by as much as a half, for the same procedure—another strong incentive to reduce federal support for training specialists. Yet, in 1979 there were only about 141,000 primary-care doctors—about 40 percent of all practicing physicians.

The Kennedy-Nixon-Mills Triangle

Interest in national health insurance during Nixon's first term, which ended in 1972, was strong, but there was too much in the way to make it possible for the idea to move forward. Medicare and Medicaid were out of control in a financial sense, and in Congress there was a strong feeling that something had to be done about this problem before serious thought could be given to a more expansive health program. Also, the government was still in the phase of enacting specialized health programs, and it would be necessary to go through a process of assimilation to see how these would work with national health insurance. During Nixon's first term, Congress had enacted several specialized health programs and expanded others that were already on the books. These, too, had to be assimilated. In the process, the administration decided it was time to move aggressively away from the categorical health progams and it proposed phasing out a number of them. Under the next administration, Gerald Ford's, this policy was refined as proposals were put forward to consolidate categorical health grants into block grants—federal monies that would go to states in large chunks to help with the cost of a broad range of health needs but with limited directives.

There were other problems that Nixon's health policy-makers believed had to be dealt with—such as the development of health care resources. It looked as if the federal programs designed to stimulate the training of more doctors and other health personnel had just about completed their task, but there were still problems; there were not enough general practitioners and there were still areas in the country that lacked an adequate supply of doctors of any kind. These shortages would have to be overcome if national health insurance were to become fully operational.

Edward Kennedy might have been thinking about how all the different pieces of health legislation he was promoting and getting Congress to enact might work to build the base for national health insurance, but it was very much frontier land and he still had a lot to learn about how it would all fit together.

In the House, Paul Rogers, the chairman of the Commerce health subcommittee, was not thinking in such global terms—he moved from one piece of special legislation to another, and from his point of view it was better to have things evolve slowly rather than start up a whole new system of health care at once. Even though Rogers's subcommittee had no direct responsibility for national health insurance—that rested, at the time, exclusively in the House with Ways and Means—his view nevertheless was influential.

Besides, as noted, the national health insurance proposals on the table aside, Congress as well as the administration was concerned about Medicare and Medicaid and there was the feeling something had to be done here. The effort to do something started in 1970 and was finally completed in 1972 when significant changes were made to those programs as part of a package of amendments to the Social Security Act.

As the 1972 amendments became law they put some clamps on the program designed to hold down cost increase. They put limits on what could be spent under Medicare for nursing home care, they gave HEW authority to put limits on the cost of basic hospital services such as room and board costs, and by creating the professional standard review organization program (PSRO) they attempted to come to grips with the problem of controlling both quality and cost. Under PSROs, groups of doctors would review hospital care for Medicare beneficiaries to ensure they were getting the most appropriate treatment and were not kept in the hospital longer than necessary.

But the 1972 amendments worked on the other end of the Medicare program as well. They opened it up to more people by making those eligible for disability payments under social security also eligible (after a two-year wait) for Medicare coverage, and by making virtually everyone with terminal kidney disease eligible for Medicare.

Thus, by 1973 as Nixon started his second term, there was a need to digest some of what had happened. Also, after his reelection, Nixon's support for national health insurance dissipated as he battled Watergate and a galloping inflation coupled with a rising federal deficit. He did not again immediately offer his national health insurance plan. By the time it did reappear in February 1974 it was a stronger proposal and had a much better chance of serving as the basis of legislation that would be considered seriously, but by then also Nixon's presidency was rapidly deteriorating.

The new Nixon plan, called the Comprehensive Health Insurance Plan, dealt with the shortcomings of the earlier one primarily by providing federal insurance for the poor and others who would not have insurance as a result of employment. It also set standards for health insurance programs provided by employers, made employee participation voluntary, and stipulated that, ultimately, employers would have to pay 75 percent of the cost of the insurance. Medicaid and Medicare would be expanded to become more comprehensive, with broader coverage for the poor and a broader definition of who was to be considered poor. Beneficiaries of the new program would have to pay a deductible of between $150 and $450 depending on the size of the family before they would start getting coverage, and then they would have to pay 25 percent of all costs, unless they were classified as poor, in which case the deductibles and coinsurance would be geared to their income. Catastrophic health insurance would be provided; when a beneficiary experienced a very expensive illness, all costs would be covered after the patient paid out $1,500.

In the meantime, interest in national health insurance was increasing in other quarters. Democrats saw the opportunity to dominate the legislative agenda as Nixon's presidency went downhill, and NHI was one proposal they wanted to push. But to win enactment of NHI in 1974 Kennedy would have to gain both the interest and support of Wilbur Mills, who still was the chairman of the House Ways and Means Committee, and to do that he would have to compromise on his own plan. This would cause problems, for as Nixon's White House unraveled, Democrats and organized labor became increasingly optimistic about the prospects of substantial victory in the fall's congressional elections. That possibility argued for no legislative compromise in 1974; wait until the next year when Democrats would dominate Congress even more heavily.

On the other hand, if they could build momentum for national health insurance that year, they might possibly, with rising public support for congressional leadership in the formulation and execution of public policy, pass it. If not, enactment would clearly be a possibility in 1975.

Other political forces were underway as the Nixon presidency declined, and of course foremost among these was the presidential election of 1976. Ted Kennedy, perennially a presidential aspirant since the death of his brother Bobby Kennedy in 1968, was clearly a contender for the 1976 nomination, if he chose to be, but others were making noises about a race as well. Among these was Wilbur Mills.

Mills was absent from work for some of the time during the early months of 1974, having been hospitalized with a back ailment. During that period, the second-ranking Democrat, Al Ullman of Oregon, took over as acting chairman of the Ways and Means Committee. And, as it happened, there was increasing discomfort during this period among Democrats in the House generally and particularly among those on the Ways and Means Committee with the autocratic way Mills had been running the panel. There were no subcommittees, and Mills had kept a tight rein over the legislative agenda, largely dictating committee activities on a day-to-day basis. House Democrats were rebelling against this autocracy, and a movement was underway to strip the committee of its authority over national health insurance and give it to the House Commerce Committee, which already had jurisdiction over most other health issues.

Ullman, the acting chairman in the early months of 1974, in an effort to head off that move said he would hold hearings on national health insurance in the spring. About that time Mills returned to work, prepared to go along with the new agenda. In fact, Mills was ready to go further, for he had already gotten together with Kennedy to develop a national health insurance plan.

In early 1974 Mills could see the end of his congressional career. He had been in Congress since 1939 and chairman of Ways and Means since 1959. It had been a demanding career and he had worked extremely hard at it. He was, everyone agreed, the master legislator, and it was a startling experience to watch him shepherd a piece of complicated legislation through a House debate and vote. He invariably did a superb job. Now he was tired; probably even he did not know how tired he was. He had watched other men become president and he believed he was as qualified. But the top spot on the Democratic ticket, as a practical matter, was not available to him. If Kennedy ran, and in early 1974 it looked as if he would, Mills as a conservative from Arkansas could provide an appropriate balance to the ticket. One way to develop that possibility was to work out a national health insurance proposal they could jointly support. Kennedy's Health Security Act was not that measure; for Mills it was too encompassing and involved too big a federal financial commitment.

The opportunity to pursue this course came to Mills in the fall of 1973 when both he and Kennedy were to participate in a St. Louis seminar with Wilbur Cohen, the guru of federal health legislation, who had served President Johnson both as an assistant secretary in HEW, where he had responsibility for shepherding through Medicare and Medicaid, and later as secretary of the department. Prior to the 1973 meeting, Mills, who already had expressed an interest in becoming a 1976 presidential contender, was making comments about the need for more federal support for health care. These had been noted by Kennedy's staff. Cohen was alerted to Mills's emerging interest, and when the three were together on the panel in St. Louis, Cohen made some remarks about the desirability of the Democratic Party having a unified position on national health insurance. Mills agreed and suggested that he and Kennedy set about doing just that. What followed was a series of meetings between Mills and Kennedy.

Those working on the Kennedy-Mills plan knew a great deal about what was going on within the administration at that time regarding development of a revised Nixon national health insurance bill, and thus they were able to take this into consideration. Mills, a fiscal conservative, was firm in the position that any Kennedy-Mills bill should cost no more than the forthcoming revised Nixon bill. The essence of the difference would be that this bill would provide a better way of doing the job. By April 2, 1974, the two men were ready to release their new plan.

The proposal was a step backward for Kennedy from the Health Security Act he had sponsored since 1971 with the blessing of organized labor. The new Kennedy-Mills bill built upon the existing Medicare program. The basic Medicare program would be retained while a new and similar program would be created for everyone else. Benefits under both programs would also be liberalized. In a significant departure from the Health Security Act, one that would cause serious problems with labor, beneficiaries would be required to pay part of the cost of treatment (a $150 deductible for up to two family members and 25 percent coinsurance), up to $1,000, after which all costs would be covered. The program would be financed by a payroll tax, similar to the Medicare tax. There would be no role for insurance companies in the basic program beyond that of serving as fiscal intermediaries, or the bill payers in behalf of the federal government as they were in Medicare. But insurance companies could sell supplementary health insurance policies to pick up where the federal insurance left off. The measure had a projected cost similar to the new Nixon bill, according to the two sponsors, but the out-of-pocket expenses for beneficiaries would be less.[62]

The major differences between this bill and Kennedy's original proposal, the Health Security Act, was that it required beneficiaries to pay some of the cost of care, whereas under his original bill virtually all essential care would be paid for by the plan. It also abandoned the concept of a nationwide health budget.

The new measure seriously strained the relationship between Kennedy and organized labor. No longer under the control of Walter Reuther, the leadership was not there to pull the union along with changes that would be necessary to win congressional enactment of national health insurance. Some of the changes in the new version, such as cost sharing and the lack of really tough controls over the health care industry, were unacceptable to labor. Within two weeks of the April 2 announcement, organized labor made clear its commitment to the original bill and its resolve to not go along with Kennedy and Mills in their new joint venture. This was a blow to Mills, who had counted on Kennedy's ability to keep labor in line and thus control important votes on the Ways and Means Committee.

In part, the intransigence of organized labor flowed from its belief that the elections in the fall of 1974 would bring in a Congress with enough Democrats to enact the original Health Security Act. Kennedy argued they had misread their crystal ball and that compromise now was better than waiting, so he decided to go ahead without labor, hoping that he could bring labor along later.[63]

Kennedy viewed the new proposal as being sufficiently attractive to win substantial support in a period when the administration was incapable of exercising much influence. What he did not know at that time was that Mills, like Nixon, was on his way out as a prominent political figure.

After the joint venture was announced in April, hearings were held in the House over the next several months. At the same time, talks were held between emissaries of Kennedy, Mills and Nixon on ways to strike a compromise. But the principals were not able to come to an agreement that could win sufficient support of the Ways and Means Committee membership. Although there was a little activity in the Senate during this period, as Russell Long talked about having the Finance Committee get down to work on his catastrophic health insurance proposal, Mills was clearly in the driver's seat. Everyone was looking to the Ways and Means Committee to take the first definitive action.

Not only was Kennedy unable to keep labor from bolting at the start, he was also unable to bring it back into the fold later on. Without labor and the political backing it provided, Kennedy lost a lot of his political appeal to Mills, and Mills was subsequently to drop Kennedy as an ally in this effort. Mills was relying on Kennedy to keep labor's supporters on the Ways and Means Committee in line when the votes were being taken, and if he wasn't going to be able to do that Mills would have to cut whatever other deal he could.

There were several reasons for Kennedy's inability to keep labor in line. His staff, largely inexperienced in high-pressure presidential politics, thought that once agreement was reached with Mills labor would not be a problem, and the staff was to some extent a reflection of Kennedy's political sophistication at that point. Although Kennedy by 1974 had been in the Senate for twelve years and had won three elections, he had, in one sense, had an easy time of it politically. Despite all the tragedy in his and his family's life, he himself had not had to work to win the mantle of presidential contender; it had been laid before him whether or not he wanted it. Thus, the assumption by him and by his staff that they could assume labor's support was easy to understand. But other things were happening in that quarter. Since Reuther's death, the UAW had become increasingly bureaucratized, and it was not easy for it to shift away from its dearly held position.

Once Kennedy's liaison with labor fell apart, he realized it was now more than ever important to bring the administration into the agreement, and so as Ways and Means was holding hearings on national health insurance during the spring of 1974, representatives of Kennedy, Mills and Caspar Weinberger, by then Nixon's HEW secretary, were meeting secretly in the basement of St. Mark's Church on Capitol Hill to develop another compromise plan. These meetings came to little, and ultimately, when it was clear that Kennedy could not recoup labor's support, it became a two-way effort between Mills and the administration, first the Nixon administration and then the Ford administration. Nixon, of course, was preoccupied with his crumbling life, but Weinberger, primarily through intermediaries, was able to keep on negotiating with Mills during this period.

In the meantime, on August 5, four days before Nixon resigned the presidency, Mills convened his Ways and Means Committee to see if it could draft an NHI bill, and it was to meet on and off over a period of several weeks. During this period there were a number of roll-call votes in the committee on various different bills, but they all lost by one vote, with Mills and most conservative Democrats voting along with Republicans against them.

When Ford took over the Oval Office he knew he was at the height of his prestige and that he could help only the Republicans, who were certain to have a hard time in that November's elections, if he diffused the national health insurance effort. If a program was enacted, then Republicans could take credit; if it failed, the blame could be put on the Democrats, since they dominated Congress. Thus, he pushed for enactment.

In a speech to a joint session of Congress on August 12, 1974, a few days after becoming president, Ford said Nixon's health insurance plan was a good program. "Why don't we write," he asked, "a good health bill onto the books in 1974, before Congress adjourns?"[64] Ford urged Weinberger to achieve a compromise with Mills, and he sought to bring Republicans along toward that end. But the American Medical Association was lobbying hard against the enactment of any NHI program, and it was successful in persuading GOP members of the Ways and Means Committee to vote against any such legislation.

By August 16, Mills realized he would have to compromise further if he was to win committee support for a bill. After a weekend of work, Mills on Monday, August 19, set the new compromise before the committee. This new version very closely resembled the (now Ford) administration's proposal.[65] Once that happened, Mills irrevocably lost the support not only of Kennedy but of a large chunk of Democrats, an earlier cadre having left him and Kennedy when the Health Security Act was abandoned. What is more, in addition to Republicans being heavily lobbied by the AMA, Kennedy declared his active opposition to the new Mills compromise, saying he would defeat it in the Senate if it got that far. It would mean that Mills could not get the support he needed. Two days later, on August 21, Mills scrapped further efforts to write a national health insurance proposal when it became clear to him that he did not have the votes and that consensus on any other plan was remote. Congress soon thereafter adjourned for a summer recess.

By October, Mills had revealed himself to be an alcoholic in serious trouble—something even his closest associates had not suspected. His problem with alcohol was spread across the front pages of the nation's newspapers, and by December he had joined Nixon as a political has-been who no longer was a topic of conversation. Although he won reelection he lost the chairmanship of the Ways and Means Committee. Two years later, in 1976, he would retire from Congress.

Coincidentally, about the time Kennedy lost his role in the development of the NHI legislation Mills was to put before Ways and Means, he was also coming to the conclusion he would not be a candidate for president in 1976.

There were many reasons for this, and the memory and political ramifications of the 1969 Chappaquiddick accident were one. Another was the family responsibilities he had assumed. He was serving as a surrogate father to the children of his murdered brother Bobby, his own children were not all well and needed his attention, his wife was having problems herself with alcohol, and there was always the threat that if he ran he would become the target for an assassin's bullet. Thus on Labor Day weekend he told his family of his decision not to run. On September 23, 1974, Kennedy announced, unequivocally, that he would not be a candidate.

Mills takes the blame for not having gotten his national health insurance proposal through the House in 1974. In an interview in 1983 he said candidly that he just was not up to the task then. He said that 1973 and 1974 were complete blanks to him, that he could not remember anything that happened during those years, adding somewhat remorsefully that the 1974 NHI effort was the only time during his tenure as Ways and Means chairman that he was unable to put together the coalition necessary to get his proposal through.

Even had the legislation won approval in the House its prognosis in the Senate was questionable, although the Senate in those days was generally more liberal than the House. When the Finance Committee in 1970 had developed its Medicare-Medicaid amendments, it added to the measure a provision that would have the federal government pick up the tab for catastrophic illness—that is, an illness that cost a family more than $2,000. Although the legislation was not enacted in 1970, Russell Long, the chairman of the Finance Committee and the sponsor of the proposal, withdrew the plan from the bill as the Senate was considering the legislation because the total package had already become very expensive. The catastrophic plan was not part of the 1972 bill as it left the Finance Committee, and thereafter the idea would be considered not as part of Medicare and Medicaid but as part of national health insurance legislation.

Thus, had Mills succeeded in getting the House to pass NHI in 1974, the chances are that the Senate would have given serious consideration only to a proposal for a catastrophic plan. And that was one that Kennedy, and organized labor along with him, had pledged to thwart.

The struggle for a 1974 national health insurance bill was over, and when it came right down to it there was not enough positive support for such a plan; thus the effort collapsed. As the year had progressed, different interest groups took increasingly hard-line positions on their favorite NHI plans, more it seems for defensive reasons than out of the conviction that their proposal was really the best one. There has always been apprehension over enacting substantial new health programs, for no one could see clearly how the landscape might change as a result of them, and as a consequence how much of that landscape, or turf as it is generally called, they might lose. Mills had thought he could bring the Democrats along if he got close to enactment, and he told the White House it would have to bring the Republicans along. But neither had the strength to capture those residual few votes, and thus the effort failed.

Now, however, the idea of national health insurance was firmly entrenched in dogma, and became the litmus test by which a Democratic presidential candidate would be rated.

Although House Speaker Carl Albert in early 1975 claimed that national health insurance would be enacted by the newly strengthened Democratic Congress, within a few weeks Gerald Ford, who shortly after assuming the presidency had asked Congress to enact a "good" health insurance bill, said, "it is time to declare a one year moratorium on new federal spending programs."[66] As the party out of power, looking forward to the presidential election to be held the following year, anticipating that any of their numerous candidates then on the horizon would support national health insurance, Democrats abandoned further work on NHI. The anticipation of a standard bearer who would support national health insurance would, of course, be satisfied, but this would not be the end of the Democratic Party's problems with NHI.

There was to be one last NHI-type gasp before President Ford left office. Even though there was no concrete effort to push legislation creating a comprehensive national health insurance program, in response to the worsening economic situation and the number of people on the unemployment rolls, Congress early in 1975 began work on a health insurance program for the unemployed in order to take care of the estimated 6 million workers who had lost their hospitalization coverage.

The measure quickly gained substantial support from a broad segment of the public and Congress, although the administration remained steadfastly opposed. Then, as hearings and more study exposed some of the technical, equity and political difficulties of the proposal, its cadre of original supporters began to slip away. One of the staunchest original backers, organized labor, moderated its support.

In the early fall the legislation was quietly laid to rest, ostensibly the victim of an irreconcilable jurisdictional conflict between the House Ways and Means and Commerce committees. Little effort was made by all parties concerned to resolve the jurisdictional conflict. The measure fell because it was finally viewed by most principals involved as a poor piece of legislation. In addition, the measure most likely would have been vetoed by President Ford and an override of that veto would have been nearly impossible.

Similar legislation had been moving through the Senate, but without the intense jurisdictional conflict. When the House snag provided an easy excuse to back away from the proposal, House and Senate sponsors of the measure tacitly agreed to let the issue die.

Although Kennedy in 1975 went back to supporting the Health Security Act, it was more of a holding action than anything else. His inability to win enactment in 1974, or even make significant progress by having it pass one chamber, was a severe disappointment, and it was not at all clear to him then what his next move should be.

A number of things were happening that had to be assimilated. The era of specialized health programs was peaking. Further expansion of existing programs would be made, but there were many signs present that from now on the trend would be downward. The economic situation was getting more rather than less severe, and it was becoming clear that the infinite expansion of the U.S. economy and thus the federal government as a provider of services was not in the cards. President Ford was proposing substantial cutbacks in health programs and even converting some to block grants under which federal dollars would go to states in large chunks with few restrictions so that states could use them as they wished. Congress, because it was dominated by Democrats and the president was a Republican, rejected this proposal, but nevertheless there was a lot of sympathy for the idea.

Most legislators by then held the view that you could not cover the country with lots of federally sponsored and supported health centers, as had once been imagined; it was time to rethink the whole federal role in health; and thus the usefulness of the Health Security Act as a guiding light in the development of national health insurance was considerably diminished.

Kennedy was stalling for time, in a sense—the next serious effort, he imagined, over national health insurance would require different ingredients. In the meantime, probably the best he could do was minimize the deterioration of existing programs.

The Conundrum of Rising Health Care Costs

Political competition and rewards aside, what drove Kennedy, Nixon and Mills to push for enactment of national health insurance was the continued upward climb of all health care costs, and particularly hospital costs. While much else was going on in the world of federal health policy, inflation in the cost of care was increasingly the driving force behind all action. There seemed to be no way to check the rise, permanently, even after inflation outside the health area had substantially lessened.

In the meantime, the nation's health care industry was becoming so large, taking an increasingly bigger share of the total economy, that because of its size alone it would be difficult if not impossible to control. In part, this meant that different groups within the health care economy—doctors, hospitals, etc.—had substantial resources with which to influence the way public decisions were made.

Health care costs had risen over the years, for many years, for a variety of complex reasons. By 1952 they were rising faster than consumer prices generally, and with only a few exceptions they would stay higher than the consumer price index. But it was not until Medicare and Medicaid were enacted that inflation in the health care sector started causing serious concern for presidents. In 1965, the year Medicare and Medicaid became law, health care costs rose 2.8 percent. In 1966, the year the program went into effect, they rose 6.6 percent and they did not drop below that figure, except for the nearly three years Nixon's price freeze was in effect, from the summer of 1971 through the spring of 1974.

Between 1970 and 1975, the average annual inflation rate in the economy as a whole was 6.7 percent, while medical care inflation was 6.9 percent. Physician services rose 6.9 percent and hospital room costs 10.2 percent.

Between 1975 and 1980, the general annual inflation rate, as measured by the consumer price index, was 8.9 percent and medical care 9.6 percent. Physician care rose 10.1 percent and hospital room costs 12 percent.

Another way of measuring the impact of increased spending for health is the percentage of gross national product it represented. In 1950, it was 4.4 percent; in 1960, 5.3 percent; in 1970, 7.5 percent; and in 1981, 9.8 percent.

Arguments have often been made that the share of gross national product for health costs is too high, but that is merely a discretion the public wants to make, and there is no absolute. Over the years, although health care costs have risen more rapidly than the consumer price index generally, they have not always risen at a faster rate than any of the other general categories of the CPI. During the early 1970s, medical care cost rises lagged behind rises in housing, and in 1978 and 1979 food prices shot up faster than medical care. In 1979 and 1980, housing and energy prices rose faster than medical care. Besides, the rise in health care costs measured more than a higher price being charged for the same services—although it did reflect that. Health care inflation is measured by total expenditures, and clearly during this era many new medical procedures and services were becoming available which patients—and insurance companies in their behalf—could purchase. There was more available in the marketplace, and these new features often were expensive.

Medicare and Medicaid, however, were clearly exacerbating the problem of rising health care costs. Outlays for the two programs in 1968 amounted to $8 billion, accounting for 57 percent of all federal health expenditures. In 1978, the outlays for the two programs combined totaled $37.1 billion, 69 percent of all federal health expenditures of $53.9 billion. In 1981, the figures jumped to an estimated $62.3 billion, 74 percent of the government's $83.9-billion health tab.

But increases in total health care costs, those paid by the private as well as the public sector, were equally dramatic.

In 1965, the year that Medicare and Medicaid were enacted, the nation spend $42 billion on health care services and supplies. Five years later, the figure had increased by 78 percent to $74.7 billion. In 1975, the total national expenditure was $132.7 billion, and in 1981 it was $286.6 billion. If the impact of the rising cost of Medicare and Medicaid was substantial, it was compounded by the tremendous growth during the 1970s in private health insurance available to workers.

The biggest impact of the Medicare and Medicaid programs was that it shifted the burden of paying for the cost of hospital care from private insurance or the individual to the federal government. By 1981, the federal government paid for 41.3 percent of hospital care, private insurance for 33.4 percent and state and local governments for 13.1 percent. Patients, thus, paid out of their own pockets about 12 percent of all hospital costs.[67]

The standard explanation for inflation in the health care sector has always been that the nation's health care system was not responsive to the usual forces of the marketplace. Instead, a triangle consisting of the patient, doctor and insurance company insulated this economy from the usual kind of competition that traditionally results in keeping prices down—the purchaser seeking out the best deal before bringing money from his pocket to buy the commodity or service. Because these traditional forces of the marketplace had not been at work, the inflation rate of prices for health care services, and particularly of hospital prices, had been higher than the rate in the economy as a whole.

The president's Council on Wage and Price Stability (COWAPS) in a December 1976 report described the economics of health care this way:

> Unlike the supplier-consumer relationship typical of other sectors of the economy, in the medical care transaction, the primary supplier of medical services, the physician, usually determines the level of services required by the consumer, the patient. Moreover, medical services are largely paid for through a system of third party payers, insurance companies and government health programs on behalf of the patient. Often unaffected by the true extent of the costs, the consumer may tend to consume a higher level of services than if he or she were able to pay for these services directly. Hospitals, a primary provider of health services, have little incentive to provide cost efficient services because of such factors as retrospective cost reimbursement by third party payors and inefficient planning which does little to stem excess capacity and duplication of expensive facilities and equipment.[68]

In 1978, COWAPS said that physician fees had tended to rise, because of rising consumer income, anticompetitive practices of organized medicine, the growth of health insurance, Medicare and Medicaid, and changes in physician-specialty distribution. Physicians' incomes increased 230 percent between 1947 and 1965, compared to 120 percent for all workers.

At the same time, the report said, "state and local medical societies put additional upward pressures on doctor bills by discouraging both price competition among physicians and the establishment of prepaid medical group practice." The growth of insurance "exempted physicians' fees from the usual restraining effects of market forces that exist for most other consumer products and services."[69]

The COWAPS study also contended that during much of the 20th century organized medicine had successfully restricted entry into the medical profession primarily by controlling state licensing procedures and the system of medical education and that during the 1930s there was evidence that the American Medical Association sought to limit the supply of new physicians to prevent erosion of income levels.

The AMA had said physicians were violating medical ethics when they accepted compensation less than the usual fee paid for that service, or when they solicited patients. Furthermore, the AMA argued, according to the COWAPS report, that doctors also violated medical ethics when they worked for health maintenance organizations because patients were then denied free choice of physicians.

The method used by health insurers to pay for physician services, the 1978 COWAPS report added, had put pressure on the cost structure. It said that the current practice of paying the usual, customary and reasonable fee instead of paying fixed dollar amounts under a fee scheduled had contributed to the price increase. The study concluded:

> Many of the forces operating in the recent past which caused higher physician fee inflation continued to exist: lack of competitive pressures to restrain fee increases, extensive health insurance coverage, and insurance reimbursement practices which allow the physician to determine the fee and level of insurer reimbursement. . . . The combination of extensive insurance coverage removing consumer resistance to the use of high cost services, increasing incidence of physicians providing additional costly diagnostic tests to ward off malpractice suits, and an increasing number of physicians and their evidenced capability to provide additional and more costly services may portend even more rapid rates of growth in consumer outlays for medical services than are currently being experienced.[70]

These would continue to be the government's standard explanations of the problem, regardless of which party controlled the White House. But there was more to the full explanation.

The continuing rise in health care costs had to do with the place of medicine in society—the prestige with which the doctor was crowned and the expectations of most people, encouraged by politicians, that they were due the best in health care available. The public tended to demand the most expensive care as a right. Rarely, although now more so than heretofore, do patients question the actions of their doctor. They accept his or her decision and are willing to pay what it costs to receive that treatment, if they can. When the moment for intensive care arrives, the consumer wants to have the kind of health insurance that will fully protect him. As that insurance became increasingly expensive for individuals to purchase, they looked to employers to buy it for them at discount rates. While about 20 percent of the population in 1983 (other than Medicare and Medicaid beneficiaries) still did not have health insurance, most people who had health insurance got it through their work. It had become a major item in wage and contract negotiations and, consequently, a huge factor in the nation's tax scheme, because these benefits did not become part of an employee's taxable income.

Another aspect of the problem of rising health care costs, as noted, was the significant improvement in delivering health care that had occurred over the years. Health care purchased in 1980 was much different, by and large, from that which was purchased in 1970, which in turn was different from that bought in 1960. Medical care in 1980, particularly that delivered in hospitals, was likely to be much more sophisticated and effective than that provided even a half-decade earlier.

This new treatment, like most other improvements, cost more. The rise in hospital costs, therefore, represented to some extent an increase in the quantity and quality of hospital services that were part of hospital care. As Martin Feldstein, a health care economist who in mid-1982 became chairman of President Reagan's Council of Economic Advisors, argued, "reducing the rise of hospital costs . . . means curtailing the quantity of these services and thereby the quality of hospital care."[71] But others would argue that although the care available was of a higher quality, it was often used to excess. Doctors often ordered more tests than were necessary and sometimes duplicative tests. As a result, the cost of health care was unnecessarily high. But it would be impossible to measure the excessive quantity, and thus to some degree the argument would always remain speculative.

Medicare and Medicaid by themselves or even in combination with all federal health programs could not be blamed entirely for the rise in hospital costs since 1965. The rise was, instead, a product of the shifting attitude of the consumer that in large part had been brought about by the emergence of health insurance as the principal mechanism used to pay hospital bills. That health care costs, exclusive of hospitals bills, kept pretty much in step with price rises generally was due largely to the fact that insurance did not generally cover much of the cost of outpatient care. The problem, then, had to do mainly with the way health costs were insured.

First adopted in the early 1930s during the Depression, when hospitals were experiencing trouble collecting their bills, health insurance was initially designed to protect the cash flow for hospitals. At that time, the hospital industry developed what became the Blue Cross-Blue Shield programs. Although the Blues would cover the cost of some outpatient care, the primary emphasis was on care in hospitals, and the insurance industry retained that bias into the 1980s. As with all insurance programs, there had been little incentive for the underwriting companies to push for economies to keep premiums down; instead, as their losses mounted, they raised premiums. Insurance companies continued to compensate for higher hospital costs until the early 1980s, when they saw their premiums moving out of the range of affordability for many purchasers. By 1983, many were taking steps to deny payment for certain procedures, to limit how much they would pay for procedures they found acceptable and to provide incentives to patients to choose outpatient over hospital care.

By the early 1950s, health insurance, particularly hospital insurance, was widely used, and ultimately it became a very significant factor in wage contracts. Both employers and unions sought to reap the tax benefits that resulted from having health insurance a fringe benefit—and thus its costs were not taxable income to either employer or employee—rather than having the employee purchase his own coverage.

But these developments fostered the attitude that hospital care was free, and physicians sought to protect their patients from high medical costs, as well as to ensure payment of their own bills, by performing as much work as possible in the hospital. Thus, by the time Medicare and Medicaid were enacted, the health care marketplace had already been substantially transformed. It was no longer working as a traditional free market, like the purchase of automobiles or clothing, where the buyer had to make a very specific decision as to how much he wanted to spend.

Prices, at least for hospital care, as an element in this traditional formula, had been virtually eliminated.

Consequently, services purchased when a person was hospitalized were no longer a factor in the patient's mind, and neither were they usually a factor in the physician's mind. The stage was set for hospitals, at the instigation of doctors, applying procedures and tests that might not be necessary, and thus for gaining the reputation of being fat, inefficient institutions.

Furthermore, insurance companies were paying whatever was charged by hospitals. This was a principle that had been embedded in law when Medicare and Medicaid were enacted as a way of making sure that things did not change too much. This practice continued. The Medicare-Medicaid programs in 1965 were given some authority to set rates, but it was modest authority, and although in subsequent years this authority was expanded somewhat, basic changes had to be made by Congress—a longer and more politically fraught process.

Inflation figures often tend to be murky and to change frequently, and so it is in the health area, but virtually everyone, regardless of which side of the debate they were on, agreed that hospital costs, if not other health care costs, were rising at a rate significantly above the rest of the economy, and that this was not good. As the problem of hospital costs became more acute, the explanation as to the cause of the problem became more politicized. That politicization was fed, regardless of the extent to which it was justified, by government reports such as the those published by the Council on Wage and Price Stability. Doctors as the principal spokesmen for the medical care industry for many years had been criticized for their opposition to Medicare and national health insurance, but now others, particularly hospitals, were coming in for their share of the blame. Kennedy, of course, in first announcing his Health Security Act in 1971, had placed much of the blame on the health insurance industry.

In 1977, when Jimmy Carter assumed the presidency, the rhetoric took another big leap forward in intensity as Joseph Califano, Carter's first secretary of Health, Education and Welfare, lambasted the health care industry generally and hospitals in particular for high costs, high profits and general lack of social conscience. The stage was set for the argument that the only solution was government regulation of the industry.

3
THE CARTER YEARS

Jimmy Carter was the first presidential candidate of either of the two principal political parties to give national health insurance a prominent place in his campaign rhetoric. He clearly thought NHI was good politics, but he was not, personally, enthusiastic about it. He came to endorse it slowly, and somewhat reluctantly, and his ideas on national health insurance were distinctly different from those generally espoused by the Democratic Party, particularly the liberal northern wing as represented by organized labor and Ted Kennedy.

Carter started thinking about running for the presidency in 1972, and his decision to do so was made by the end of that year, although public affirmation of that decision did not come about until December 1974. In the meantime, he developed the themes on which he would run. At first, he did not seriously consider pushing a national health insurance program. Carter as governor of Georgia had developed several important state health programs, and good health care would logically be a part of the theme of his presidency. Those around him during the early days of formulating themes, however, did not stress the idea of national health insurance because of Carter's natural conservatism, and particularly because of his expressed desire not to put additional pressure on the federal budget—national health insurance, by any measure, would be expensive.

But they also knew that as a Democratic candidate, Carter would be expected, at least by some, to embrace national health insurance. As these aides surveyed the political landscape, the importance of support from organized labor, and particularly from the United Auto Workers, which strongly endorsed Kennedy's Health Security Act and perhaps was the most effective labor union politically, loomed larger and larger.

Carter would be a candidate from the South, indeed the rural South, where organized labor was not strong, and he would be running against candidates who were already known and popular in the industrial Northeast and Midwest, where the strength of labor was greatest. During this preannouncement period it became clear to Carter's aides, and to Carter himself, that he needed the support of labor to win the nomination, and in order to get that support he would have to commit himself to push for enactment of a comprehensive national health insurance program.

But if Carter needed labor, labor in turn needed him. Carter was fairly well known in the South and had the best chance of any other contender of beating former Alabama Governor George Wallace, the perennial segragationist candidate for the Democratic presidential nomination, in the crucial Florida primary. If Wallace could be knocked off in that primary, which he had won four years earlier, he might at that point be stopped from further influencing the nominating process. Supporting Carter, therefore, was the way to accomplish this objective. But the UAW wanted a quid pro quo. Thus, Carter and the UAW became important to each other.

The two camps first made contact in late 1975, at which time some preliminary discussions were held, but it was not until Carter won the Iowa caucus in January 1976 that the UAW saw him as the best candidate to bump Wallace.

The UAW leaders ideally wanted Carter to endorse the Health Security Act; it was their program and that's what they wanted, but they did not insist on Carter's endorsing the proposal completely. For his part, Carter wanted to make his commitment vague in order to retain as much flexibility as possible when he actually came to write a national health insurance plan. Thus, the two finally agreed on a set of principles, and these ultimately were set forth in an April 1976 speech to the Student National Medical Association (SNMA) in which Carter called for reforms to improve health care services and how they were financed. In that speech, he stressed the need for universal and mandatory coverage to ensure that everyone had the same level of benefits and care. He wanted to make preventive care and treatment in the early stages of illness more available. The cost of the program, he said, should be paid for by a combination of employer and employee payroll taxes and by general tax revenues. Physicians would be paid according to a fee schedule and hospitals would also be paid a set amount for a specific service. He wanted the full program phased in over a number of years. He told the SNMA audience: "As president I would want to give our people the most rapid improvement in individual health care that the nation can afford, accommodating first those who need it most, with the understanding that it will be a comprehensive program in the end."[72]

He was, in other words, going to start out with a modest program and work up to a comprehensive one.

Although the speech was made a month after the Florida primary of March 9, the basic commitment was made before that election.

In the process of negotiating the speech during the early months of 1976, Carter came, reluctantly, to accept virtually all but two of the basic ingredients of Kennedy's Health Security Act.

The only absolute reservations he made during the process were the right to include deductibles and copayments and to use the insurance industry in the proposal that he would as president finally send to Congress. These were significant reservations, for they violated basic principles of the Health Security Act and thus put a substantial gulf between Carter and the UAW and Kennedy. But they were differences Kennedy, labor and others glossed over until Carter was president.

Even though his speech called for financing by a payroll tax to be paid in part by employers and in part by employees (just as Medicare is financed), by withholding the reservation that he could use insurance companies in much the same capacity that they presently functioned—that is, underwriting the insurance—he implied that the scheme would not be wholly within the operational embrace of the federal government. Also, by withholding the possibility of including deductibles and copayments, Carter reserved an option that could be used to mitigate the cost of his program. Even though Kennedy deviated when he joined with Mills in 1974, he always had been committed to a totally federally run system and one in which there were no copayments or deductibles. What is more, Kennedy had repeatedly over the years lambasted the health insurance industry as being incompetent.

Carter was not as concerned about the philosophical aspects of a national health insurance program—committing federal resources to ensuring health care for everyone, poor and rich alike—as he was about the budgetary impact of the program. He was tremendously concerned about the rise each year of federal expenditures, and foremost in his campaign was a commitment to check that rise. National health insurance, no matter how one looked at it, undermined that commitment, and thus he found himself constantly trying to pull away from it. From time to time he reviewed the commitment embedded in the SNMA speech, and made efforts to modify some of the concepts.

In part, too, Carter by linking himself this way to the UAW's health plan was bothered about becoming too closely associated with Kennedy. From the moment Carter first decided to seek the presidency, he had eyed Kennedy as a serious challenger, and probably one he could not overcome if Kennedy ran. Kennedy's decision in the summer of 1974 not to run for the 1976 nomination freed Carter from a contest he was dreading, but another dread developed—that he, Carter, would be drawn into the vortex of Kennedy liberalism; and national health insurance became the symbol of that liberalism. It was during this period that Carter developed the attitude toward Kennedy that was to plague him through his presidency.

The UAW-Carter liaison paid off in Florida when Carter won that state's primary on March 9. That was a particularly important victory for Carter because it had pitted him against not only Wallace in the homeland of both, it came right after he was defeated in the Massachusetts primary. If Carter could not win in Florida against the perennially popular Wallace it was questionable that he could win the presidential election. Wallace had won the 1972 Florida primary with 42 percent of the vote; this time Carter was able to beat Wallace by four percentage points, with a total of 34.5 percent of the vote. A week after the Florida primary, Carter generated more momentum by winning the Illinois Democratic primary with 48 percent of the vote.

By then, Carter's campaign was rolling, and for all practical purposes national heath insurance had served its purpose. Now it became important for the UAW to endorse Carter officially for the nomination, which it did, so that Carter would not become the candidate of conservative Democrats.[73]

As the campaign progressed, Carter continued to spell out his views on national health insurance and on health issues generally.

In preparation for the Democratic Party platform, Carter on June 12 delivered a message to the platform committee that again gave what liberal Democrats and labor would take to mean a commitment to Kennedy's Health Security Act. "We need," he said, "a national health insurance program financed by general tax revenues and employer/employee shared payroll tax which is universal and mandatory. Such a program must reduce barriers to preventive care, provide for uniform standards and reforms in the health care delivery system, and assure freedom of choice in the selection of physician and treatment centers."[74] Virtually the same language was incorporated into the health plank of the Democratic Party platform adopted by the convention in July.

In a June press conference, Carter emphasized that a national health insurance program was high on his agenda: "I say that we need a national health insurance program. I mean to do it. Nobody's ever done it. . . . That will be the difference [made by my administration]."[75]

The Health Security Action Council, the Washington-based nationwide grass-roots citizens' lobby that was pushing the Kennedy-labor Health Security Act, attempted to nail the commitment home. In a June memorandum it argued that "only the Kennedy . . . bill will fit the criteria" spelled out in the Democratic Platform.[76]

But Carter still did not feel committed to or locked in by the Kennedy bill. Once president, it was made clear, he would write his own national health insurance program rather than adopt an existing proposal.

In a June 1976 interview, Peter Bourne, a psychiatrist who was in charge of candidate Carter's Washington office and who had a key role in developing Carter's initial positions on health, emphasized that Carter was committed to developing a role in NHI for the private insurance carrier—a role that was to go beyond that of serving as financial intermediary to actually underwriting the program. Such a role would ensure insurance carriers a very large stake in NHI, opening the door to substantial earnings. Bourne said: "Carter believes private insurance should be given a chance to show they can do it. If they can't do it within three to four years then the task should be taken away from them and all of the responsibility assumed by the federal government. The most important thing would be to develop an efficient system."[77]

Bourne emphasized also that Carter's national health insurance program would differ from the Kennedy bill in one other significant way: Carter's NHI program would be phased in over several years, either by groups of individuals covered (aged and young at first, other age groups later) or by service (for example, all short-term inpatient care and outpatient care first, other types of care later).

Carter as candidate was convinced that some kind of controls on the cost of health services was necessary—controls that would extend across the board. In fact, during the campaign it seemed likely that Carter's first effort at controlling health care costs would be to pick up on the proposals of the Ford administration and the Democratic Congress for placing ceilings on payments made under Medicare and Medicaid for health services, an effort that would precede enactment of NHI. In his April 1976 SNMA speech, Carter had said: "Medical care costs must be controlled. We must find incentives for productivity and efficiency. . . . Rates for institutional care and physician services should be set in advance, prospectively."[78]

But if Carter was reluctant about national health insurance because of the depth of the commitment, he didn't seem reluctant about expanding federal responsibility in other regards. As president, he said, he would seek to eliminate abuses in the delivery of health care and to improve its quality. Furthermore, Carter believed, according to Bourne, that before national health insurance was enacted there must be in place a health care delivery system that had the capacity to deliver the services that would be demanded. This was an issue that had bothered presidents as far back as Franklin Roosevelt. Carter told the black medical students: "We have built a haphazard, unsound, undirected inefficient nonsystem which has left us unhealthy and unwealthy at the same time."[79]

Then he later told the platform committee: "We must reorganize the physical plant of our health care delivery system. We need to initiate effective coordination between our physical facilities—buildings, expanding, modernizing, relocating and converting them as needed in order to provide the best possible medical care at reasonable cost."[80]

Carter also placed emphasis on the need for health care professionals who were not physicians—such as nurse practitioners and physician extenders—but who could treat people without the supervision of a physician. These people would often work in remote areas where physicians themselves were not available. He wanted registered nurses, physician assistants and other paraprofessionals to be able to deliver health care.

Carter would also invest federal dollars in a way to bring better understanding of diseases and development of systems to detect disease early. Carter said in his SNMA speech:

> First, our emphasis must be on prevention of the killers and cripplers of our people. Our purpose must be to promote health, not just to provide health care as such, and this includes initiatives in ensuring adequate family incomes and clean environment as well as reforming the financing of health care. Reform of the welfare morass may prevent more sickness and disease during the next generation than could be achieved by placing $600,000 body scanning x-rays in every hospital.[81]

Carter also looked to the development of more systems of health care. He said he would strengthen the network of community health and mental health centers and health maintenance organizations—systems that made it possible for people to get all the care they needed in one place.

As the 1976 campaign progressed, Carter emphasized repeatedly that national health insurance could come only after he had reached his goal of a balanced budget.

In an interview in *Playboy*, published in that magazine's November 1976 issue, Carter became more explicit in his views on NHI and in doing so drove the wedge between himself and Kennedy's Health Security Act even deeper.

When asked by *Playboy* why he did not support the Kennedy bill, Carter made it clear that he preferred a nongovernmental system to the fullest extent possible. "Whenever the private sector can perform a function as effectively and efficiently as the government," he said, he preferred to "keep it within the private sector."[82]

Once the election was over, national health insurance got pushed to the rear of the Carter domestic program, even though it continued to remain nominally an important item.

Immediately, Carter's economic advisors argued that a national health insurance program would be too expensive an undertaking for a new president who had won, as most of those advisors saw it, on economic issues. New people were brought in to help with the transition and the task for some would be to develop health policy. Joseph Onek, a young lawyer who had worked on health issues for public interest groups, headed the health task force in the transition and he immediately saw the need for a device to check rising hospital costs before a more ambitious national health insurance program was undertaken. Thus, the plan for Carter's hospital cost containment program was born, and it would be the only major health initiative developed during the transition.

Once president, Carter indicated that he planned by the end of 1977, his first year in office, to have a scheme for implementing his national health program and reiterated the need for a phased-in approach. He would, he said later, send details of the plan to Congress in early 1978, but in the meantime his priority was to get health care costs under control.

The Other Pieces of Carter's Health Policy Agenda

Like every president, Carter had to articulate his health policy through his budget, and although Gerald Ford, by the time Carter was inaugurated, had already presented Congress with the budget for the upcoming fiscal year, Carter in late February 1977 sent his own budget plan forward. The important aspects, as far as health issues were concerned, carried changes in federal health policy beyond budget amounts. In addition to announcing that legislation would soon be proposed to contain inflation in hospital costs, the Carter budget message said that two other health proposals were being readied. One would provide for reimbursement under Medicare for services delivered in health clinics serving poor or rural areas by paraprofessionals, physician assistants, nurses and other health care professionals who were not physicians when not working under the direct supervision of medical doctors. It was a significant and even radical departure from existing policy. The other proposal would provide for a comprehensive health program for children, which became known affectionately as CHAP (for child health assessment program). CHAP, although it was the most creative health bill other than NHI to be put forward by Carter during his four years in the White House, still remained a proposal when he left office.

The first proposal, however, with some modifications, became law rather quickly. Before its enactment, Medicare regulations required that reimbursements could be made only for services provided by or under the direct supervision of a physician, which meant that a physician had to be present at the location. The change was offered as a way of making health clinics that serve rural or city poverty areas eligible for reimbursement for treatment provided to Medicare beneficiaries. Although the initial cost of the proposal was modest—approximately $25 million the first year—the ramifications for national health insurance were broad, for one of the issues any NHI plan had to deal with was whether to continue the practice of having physicians ultimately responsible for health care, and thus the conduit through which all reimbursement flowed. If services under NHI were covered only when provided under the direct supervision of a physician, as suggested by the Medicare prototype, then the demand on medical practitioners once NHI began could be overwhelming. But if nonphysicians could deliver services under the program, then the adequate availability of care became more possible. The issue was important not only in insuring the availability of adequate health care personnel in remote areas, but also in checking the rise in health prices, for the cost of care delivered by a physician was more expensive than when delivered by a nurse practitioner. Enactment of the proposal was an important step in developing the basis for a successful national health insurance program, although as a practical matter it had a very limited impact.

But if Carter's initial health policy had some creative twists to it, like virtually all other domestic policy its potential for success was grounded in the dollar requests, and here the new president was to be nearly as cautious as his predecessors. Like virtually every other recent president, Carter came to the presidency expressing above all else a concern for the integrity of the federal budget, and pledged to balance that budget by the end of his term. This concern permeated all his decisions on domestic issues. Nowhere was the concern more evident than in the area of health.

With Carter focusing on ways to curtail the escalation of health care costs, particularly those of hospitals, it soon became clear that he was not prepared to increase the level of federal investment in the health care system until that escalation was checked.

Thus, Carter's February 1977 recommendations for federal health spending in fiscal 1978, which would begin the following October, were essentially the same as President Ford had offered a few weeks earlier. Only where he was requesting a few special initiatives, such as alternatives to abortion and better health care for children (the CHAP program), did Carter propose spending more in fiscal 1978 than in the previous fiscal year.

Constituencies of federal programs as well as some congressional leaders were severely disappointed if not angered by the Carter health budget. Repeatedly during the Nixon-Ford years, Congress had added more to the health budget than had been proposed by the administration. Once the legislation had been given initial congressional approval, it was often necessary for Congress to assert itself again by overriding a veto. There had thus been hope that, as a Democrat, Carter would change that trend and propose a level of federal spending for health programs that would at least halt the decomposition of these programs begun as a result of the Nixon-Ford policies.

Cutbacks in appropriations for health programs during the Nixon-Ford years had meant that those programs had grown much more slowly than originally anticipated and that some did not grow at all, but shrank instead. Curtailment in federal spending for health meant that community health centers, for example, had to find money elsewhere, and if they could not find any they had to curtail services or perhaps go out of business. When services were curtailed, the first to go were those aimed at maintaining good health, such as early treatment for minor illnesses, and the last to go were the services for the very sick. This drift seriously undercut the foundation for comprehensive health care that Edward Kennedy and others who wanted a program of national health insurance were trying to construct.

A rise in federal spending in 1977, it was hoped, would afford those programs the opportunity to stabilize and perhaps be strengthened to better serve as the underpinning for national health insurance. But a significant boost in federal health spending, except where mandated by law for Medicare and Medicaid, would not occur under Carter.

The Struggle to Cap Hospital Costs

When Carter entered the White House, Congress already had on its docket legislation designed to dampen rising hospital costs, but only as they affected Medicare and Medicaid. The Medicare-Medicaid Administrative Reform Act was sponsored by Senator Herman Talmadge, a Democrat from Georgia, who through 1980 was chairman of the Senate Finance health subcommittee, which had jurisdiction over the two programs. The genesis of the measure had occurred several years earlier in response not only to rising Medicare and Medicaid costs but in anticipation of a larger federal role in health, perhaps through national health insurance or a totally federally run Medicaid program. The Talmadge bill would control Medicare and Medicaid costs by using a series of administrative reforms and incentives to keep costs down. The core of the bill was a device to reward hospitals whose routine operating costs were below the average while penalizing hospitals whose operating costs were substantially above average. But the proposal went further—it gave incentives to physicians to accept the fee allowed by Medicare as the full amount for providing the care and thus not charge the patient more than the standard 20 percent copayment. The Talmadge bill also gave doctors incentives to perform surgery in their offices rather than in hospitals.

The chief weakness of the Talmadge bill was that it applied only to the Medicare and Medicaid programs. Although, if it worked as anticipated once it was enacted, it would have put a check on federal expenditures through Medicare and Medicaid, it would not have touched the cost of care paid for through private insurance policies.

Joe Onek, who led the health policy task force of Carter's transition team and later was the chief White House staff person for health issues, during the interregnum talked on numerous occasions with congressional health leaders, and their message was that inflation was the most worrisome health issue; they wanted it brought under control before they would consider any expansion of federal responsibility for health care. This prompted Onek to urge the development of hospital cost-containment legislation. Although the initial bias may have been to go forward with the Talmadge Medicare-Medicaid proposal, further examination led Onek to conclude that its enactment would only exacerbate the problem. The Carter administration argued that because of this limitation, the Talmadge proposal would not dampen hospital inflation overall—only in relation to Medicare and Medicaid. The result would be a ballooning of costs for non-Medicare- and non-Medicaid-supported health care services—the Medicare-Medicaid cost shift that the Republican minority of the House Ways and Means Committee had anticipated in 1965 as Medicare was being enacted. The Carter administration would then be accused, and with some justification, of shifting the burden of controlling rising health care costs to others to save on federal expenditures.

Thus, the decision was made to spread the burden and go for caps on all hospital costs.

Carter first announced his hospital cost-containment plan as a major piece of domestic legislation in the spring of 1977, to a cool reception by

Congress and a hostile reaction by the medical industry, particularly hospitals. The congressional reaction was a surprise since it was the first time that the Democratic Congress had had a Democrat in the White House in eight years, and because it was one of Carter's first legislative proposals.

This cool reception also surprised Carter's health policy-makers because they had been led to believe by members of Congress that legislation along these lines would be well received. They thought it would move rapidly once the measure came to Capitol Hill, but Congress was made wary by the strong initial negative reaction of the hospital industry, which maintained that the proposal was merely a repackaging of Nixon's price controls. Each member of Congress had at least one hospital in his home community, and on its board sat several influential members of that community, so the views of the hospital industry were given careful attention on Capitol Hill. The hospital industry argued that the proposal was unnecessary and would be destructive to a health care system already overburdened with federal regulation.

There were two main reasons for Carter to ask for enactment of the hospital cost-containment proposal. First, as noted, was the need, as he made explicit, to reduce the high rate of inflation in hospital costs. The second reason—less visible but perhaps more important in a political context—was that the deficits of Carter's budgets were tempered when his budget-makers included anticipated savings from hospital cost containment. Carter's first budget carried a proposed deficit of nearly $60 billion, but it would have been several billion dollars higher without the projected savings from hospital cost containment. While Carter estimated lower budget deficits as his term went on, hospital cost containment continued to be an important ingredient in paring federal expenditures overall. The hospital cost-containment plan would, the new president argued, result in substantial savings to both the general public and the federal government. Once fully effective, it would save as much as $60 billion over five years in public and private expenditures from all sources, $25 billion of which would be savings in federal expenses. Later, in Reagan's tenure the Carter budget deficits would seem highly desirable compared to the actual size of the current deficits. But back in those days deficits of the magnitude Carter was dealing with were still considered a serious political liability. Thus did hospital cost containment get drawn right into the middle of presidential politics.

The Carter administration argued that legislation to control hospital costs was necessary because traditional forces of the marketplace would not keep hospital costs down. The Carter economics team was strongly pushing deregulation for the rest of the economy—particularly the airlines—but reversed course 180 degrees when it came to hospitals.

Even though the health policy leaders in Congress had strongly suggested that they would be receptive to hospital cost containment and would embrace it once it came forward, they probably then, in late 1976, were not fully aware themselves of how their institution, Congress, had changed. By the mid-1970s many federal health programs—as well as others—had become more heavily enshrouded in regulation, which was in part a product of congressional reaction to Nixon's attempts to administer federal programs in ways that resulted in their dismantlement. Greater regulation accomplished its immediate objective of thwarting Nixon's policies, but in the long run it placed a greater burden on those throughout the land—in this case hospitals and other health care facilities—that were the recipients of aid from the federal programs. Now they had to cope with the regulations. They began reacting to this burden, and the first to hear their concerns were their representatives and senators.

By the time Carter entered the White House, this concern was being well articulated. Thus Congress, when it came right down to it, was not so sure it wanted to regulate so heavily the hospital industry—and the hospital industry did what it could to solidify that attitude.

The hospital cost-containment legislation had other obstacles to overcome. It was all stick and no carrot, as Stuart Eizenstat described it in a 1983 interview—it hit hospitals over the head and offered no incentives, nothing positive, in return. Furthermore, there was really no constituency for the legislation. People throughout the land understood, intellectually, that hospital inflation was high, and they were against this in theory, but in practice, in most cases, the high inflation rate did not affect them directly, only indirectly through higher health insurance premiums, and many people had these partially or totally paid for by their employers. What is more, when they had to go to the hospital they wanted the best care possible, and if federal regulation of hospital costs meant cutting back on the quality of care they personally would receive then they would have doubts about the federal program.

But perhaps more than anything else, it was the resemblance of the Carter hospital cost-containment package to the last version—called Phase IV—of the Nixon wage and price control scheme that set Congress against the measure. The experience of wage and price controls from mid-1971 into the spring of 1974 had been a bitter one for the health care industry. When the controls were first instigated they applied to all segments of the economy, but by the end of 1973 the Nixon administration was ready to lift these controls from all areas except the health care and petroleum industries, and in the case of health care the administration wanted to make the controls more stringent than they had been. With all controls due to expire in the spring of 1974, the Nixon administration asked Congress to renew its authority, a request that Congress ignored. But before the authority lapsed, the administration was able to implement briefly the fourth phase of the price-control plan, which held increases in hospital revenues to 7.5 percent a year.

These new controls in 1974 had caused many problems for hospitals, but perhaps most important was their potential for pitting hospital administrator against the physicians who practiced in the hospital and thus were the hospital's access to income—it was they who brought in the business. Since hospitals were to be limited in how much they could increase their revenue each year, it might be necessary for administrators to tell the physicians to limit the services they wanted to provide to patients. That was not an acceptable practice to either party. The issue was mooted when the price-control scheme was allowed to die, and following the subsequent lifting of controls, hospital prices, as well as health care prices generally, again began to rise dramatically.

Now, in 1977, once the Carter administration's new hospital cost-containment proposal reached Capitol Hill, most legislators who had been there during the earlier period saw little difference between the Nixon-Ford plan and the new Carter proposal. When this similarity became clear, Congress gave the proposal a cool reception.

Joe Califano, Carter's HEW secretary, became very dedicated to winning enactment of the hospital cost-containment legislation. Some attributed Califano's zeal to his generally combative nature and the opportunity to paint a large industry as the bad guys ripping off the consumer. Others suggested that it was simply his ambition to pursue liberal Democratic dogma by placing a big chunk of the economy under federal regulation.

In any case, he was extremely critical of the hospital industry, and of doctors as well, for what he described as reaping excessive profits. And this criticism quickly became an obstacle to achieving a middle course. Califano repeatedly used terms like "bloated" and "fat" to describe hospitals and implied that doctors, by earning such high salaries, were not performing in the public interest. This, despite the fact that reports he filed on his income from his law practice as he entered the cabinet showed that in 1976 he had earned $505,000—fees that for the most part were deducted by the businesses that retained him, thus reducing by that amount their taxable earnings. Califano missed the point entirely when, in his 1981 book describing his experience in the Carter cabinet, he tried to pass off his 1976 income by noting that he had paid $276,000 that year in income taxes.[83]

Califano was a controversial figure from his first days in the Carter cabinet until he was fired in the summer of 1979. His first experience in government had been as a young man during the early days of the Kennedy administration when he served—as one of the so-called whiz kids—in the Department of Defense as an aide to Secretary Robert McNamara. Later, when Lyndon Johnson became president, Califano moved to the White House where he became the chief aide for domestic matters. His memoirs, *Governing America: An Insider's View from the White House and the Cabinet,* reflects a warmer feeling for his days in the Johnson White House than in the Carter cabinet. And surely what he learned at the White House colored the way he carried out his job at HEW. While at the White House he was known to sometimes handle cabinet officers roughly, and once in the cabinet he became very aggressive, sometimes ignoring directives from White House staff and pursuing his own agenda. After awhile, the White House aides closest to Carter, such as Hamilton Jordan and Jody Powell, saw Califano more as their foe than as their ally. At one point, early in the Carter administration, Califano told Stuart Eizenstat, who was Carter's chief aide for domestic issues, that he recalled how he, Califano, when he had Eizenstat's job, had pushed around cabinet officers and that he wasn't going to let the Carter White House staff treat him that way.[84]

There were other problems created by Califano, problems resulting from the basic ingredient in all political action, the chemistry between individuals. Califano could be a difficult person to work with, and this compounded the problems for hospital cost containment. He often did not communicate well with principals on Capitol Hill, both elected members and their staffs, choosing instead to provide them with his positions on a take-it-or-leave-it basis. Too often, Hill staffers found that a Califano emissary would arrive in their offices with a proposal regarding hospital cost containment, or another piece of health legislation, and present it as the last word.

Califano wanted it that way, though. He sought to keep not only his adversaries, but also his allies—the White House staff and members of Congress—on the defensive, or at least somewhat in the dark as to what he was doing. He kept his plans and recommendations under wraps until the last possible moment, so that when they did go forward to either the White House or Capitol Hill, those who had to pick them up had a limited amount of time to react—and develop an alternative. This technique was one of the things that made it possible for him to have near-total control over development of policy for which he had responsibility. Another was his mastery of the issues and the problems—he often knew more about the subject than anyone else, at least outside of his department.

The stress became particularly acute between Califano's department and the Finance Committee, which in the Senate largely determined the fate of hospital cost containment as well as other major health legislation. There the principal staff person for health matters was Jay Constantine, who had many of Califano's personality traits: he was arrogant, stubborn and smart. What is more, as the Carter administration came into office, Constantine made no secret of his desire to be named to the newly created HEW job of inspector general, the internal watchdog on fraud and abuse in the department. But Califano would not give Constantine serious consideration, so he stayed on at his job with the committee where he was to have a determining influence over all Carter's most important health proposals.

Califano attributes the problems of hospital cost containment in part to another personality clash—one between him and Dan Rostenkowski, who in 1977 and 1978 was chairman of the Ways and Means health subcommittee. Califano suggests in his memoirs that when he refused to appoint a Rostenkowski protégé to an HEW job in Chicago, Rostenkowski's home town, Rostenkowski retaliated by pushing a version of hospital cost containment that gave the hospitals a chance, before federal regulations became effective, to cut inflation voluntarily. This was a position the Carter administration opposed in 1977. Califano says that when Rostenkowski did that, "our bill was dead in the House Ways and Means Committee"—but he failed to recognize that Rostenkowski paved the way for a compromise and the version Carter would support in 1979.[85]

Throughout the entire effort surrounding hospital cost containment, the battle against it was led, and increasingly so, by David Stockman, a Republican representative from Michigan and later Reagan's director of the Office of Management and Budget. During the Carter years, Stockman was a member of the House Commerce Committee, and when in the summer of 1978 the full committee was debating the measure, Stockman led the attack against it. During the last two years of Carter's term, Stockman joined the health subcommittee as well, where he continued his opposition from a more strategic spot. Stockman, an articulate person who understood federal programs very well, gave the opposition its intellectual elegance and was able crisply to point out the proposal's shortcomings—that it was an exceedingly clumsy program that would be exceedingly difficult to administer.

There were two reasons for limiting the cost-containment program to hospitals rather than extending it to cover the entire health care industry. First, hospitals had the highest level of inflation and 40 percent of their income came from the federal government. Second, they were an easily identifiable and relatively manageable group, in terms of exercising control, for they all made reports to HEW under Medicare, and there were only about six thousand in the country.

Physicians in private practice, by contrast, got a relatively small proportion, on the average, of their income from Medicare and Medicaid, and there was no standardized mechanism for having them report to HEW. Physicians would be a harder group to tackle. Thus, no serious thought was given to placing their fees under control. But that decision laid the administration open to a contradiction—why regulate only part of the health care economy, particularly when doctors by and large determine hospital treatment?

Carter at first called his cost-containment proposal a transitional effort until a more comprehensive program could be designed—presumably what became his national health insurance plan. The initial proposal sought to limit price increases by community hospitals, which provided acute care rather than long-term care, to 9 percent in the first year and lesser amounts in subsequent years. The measure also sought to limit expenditures for new capital equipment and construction for community hospitals.

The program would be enforced by requiring hospitals to pay an excise tax of 150 percent of the amount in excess of the cost limitation. Third-party payers—that is, insurance companies—who paid fees in excess of the limit to any hospital would be taxed on the excess paid.

The proposal limited wage increases for hospital workers, but here, very early in the game, the Carter people had to make a huge concession. In order to get organized labor to go along with the plan, blue-collar workers in hospitals were to be exempted from these limits. This provision set the precedent of further exemptions, and as the legislation wandered through Congress these exemptions grew—and grew—until fewer hospitals were to be covered than were exempted by the legislation.

Because of its sweeping nature that overlapped existing congressional committee boundaries, the cost-containment legislation had to be considered by several panels. In the House, the measure went before the Interstate and Foreign Commerce and the Ways and Means committees, and their health subcommittees. In the Senate, both the Labor and Human Resources and Finance committees shared jurisdiction.

As hearings on the proposal were held in both the House and Senate in late spring of 1977, it became clear that, even if it were to get anything at all, the administration could never get its full package. But this was a compromise Carter's health people were a long time accepting, and in the end their stubbornness was a major reason for the failure of the legislation. Had they made in the beginning the concessions they finally made in the end, they might well have won enactment of the proposal, capitalizing on the strong momentum of a new president in his first year supported by a Congress dominated by his own party.

There was little action on the hospital cost-containment proposal in 1977. In the Senate, the Human Resources Committee approved the measure after its health subcommittee, led by Kennedy, built in some modest modifications. From there, however, the measure had to go to the Finance Committee before it could go to the floor, and in that panel, both its chairman, Russell Long, and Herman Talmadge, who chaired the health subcommittee, were predisposed to Talmadge's Medicare-Medicaid reform bill.

In the House, Paul Rogers was able to win approval of the measure, again with some modifications, in his health subcommittee, but Rostenkowski's Ways and Means health subcommittee did not act on the proposal.

The next year, then, 1978, was to be the big year for hospital cost containment.

The first stop was to be the full Commerce Committee. The effort to win approval of hospital cost containment was to be Paul Rogers's swan song. Before the committee completed action on the measure in July, Rogers announced that he would retire at the end of the year.

It was, in a way, a curious move, for Rogers, well respected and well liked both in the full House and in the committee, was in line to become chairman. Although Rogers was still several seats away in seniority from the chairman's seat, he might well have hurdled over the gap to become chairman when Harley Staggers, then chairman, retired two years later. In any case, in the early summer of 1978, in time to open up his seat in the forthcoming Florida primary, Rogers told a surprised audience that he would not run again. He said that he looked forward to more lucrative pastures and a different kind of professional life.

Although the announcement of his retirement came in the midst of a frustrating legislative effort, it also came at a time, as he acknowledged in an interview five years later, when the job of being responsible for much of the health legislation in Congress had shifted from designing and creating new programs that could have an impact on the nation's health care system to a holding action and in fact a retrenchment. The federal government was by 1978 attempting to withdraw somewhat from its involvement in health issues.[86]

The debate in the Commerce Committee in 1978 stretched over more than a month. Numerous amendments were offered, and most won or lost by a vote or two.

Tempers flared as the committee worked on drafting the legislation, and arms were twisted. Tim Lee Carter, the ranking Republican on the health subcommittee and a physician himself, said at one point that he had been turned against the bill, which he originally supported, because of the way it was being loaded down with compromises and favors to gain votes. He cited the agreement by the administration to exempt from the cap on hospital expenses wage increases for hospital workers, an effort that he correctly characterized as a blatant attempt to win the support of labor, and an agreement to build a new veterans hospital in Camden, N.J., in order to win the support of that city's representative in Congress, Democrat James Florio.

The crucial vote in the committee came on July 18, and it was one the administration expected to win. But Marty Russo, a Chicago Democrat, who the administration had thought would vote with it—in fact to be the deciding vote in their favor—instead voted with opponents of the bill, thus killing it by a one-vote margin, 22–21. The vote was on an amendment to remove the mandatory provisions of the bill and make it entirely voluntary. There was a big flurry when the defeat was realized, for Russo, a product of Chicago's well-disciplined ward politics, was not usually seen as a particularly bright or independent fellow, and here he was voting against not only the leader of his party, the president, but against his mentor, his fellow Democrat from Chicago and chairman of the Ways and Means health subcommittee, Dan Rostenkowski, whom all recognized as a shrewd politician and an able leader when he wanted to be. Following the vote, Rogers, who was leading the effort to win approval, took Russo into the back room, where efforts were made to get him to switch, but to no avail. When they returned, Russo declined to change his vote, thus allowing the defeat to stand. It was an incident that led cynics to remark that Rostenkowski was really against the bill, for surely Russo had told him in advance how he would vote and Rostenkowski, they believed, could have talked him out of it had he wanted to.

In the House, the proposal had to be considered as well by the Ways and Means Committee. Earlier, in 1978, that panel's health subcommittee had approved a plan that its chairman, Dan Rostenkowski, previously had urged upon the hospital industry. He had suggested that hospitals pursue a voluntary effort to cut the increase in costs by 2 percent in 1978 and another 2 percent in 1979. Administration officials had denigrated the proposal, arguing that if successful at all it would be due only to the threat of federal legislation and that a voluntary effort would never work in the long run. The legislation ultimately reported by Rostenkowski's subcommittee combined the voluntary approach, which by then had been adopted by the industry, with the mandatory program advocated by the administration—if inflation could not be reduced two percentage points a year by voluntary action, then federal controls would be triggered. Once the legislation was defeated in the Commerce Committee, the Ways and Means Committee put it aside until the Senate acted.

The last round in the struggle for 1978 was set for the full Senate when it took up the Medicare-Medicaid reform act, the Talmadge bill.

As that bill went to the floor in the last days of the 1978 session, it did not carry any of the administration's program. The Finance Committee, before it cleared the bill in early August, had considered the administration's proposal, but rejected it by a 9–7 roll-call vote. The measure as reported thus applied only to hospital bills paid by Medicare and Medicaid.

Gaylord Nelson, then a Democratic senator from Wisconsin and the administration's chief ball carrier in the Senate and on the Finance Committee on hospital cost containment, had offered an amendment to the Talmadge bill patterned after Rostenkowski's proposal—the administration's mandatory program would become effective only if the industry's voluntary program failed to reduce inflation. Nelson, when he lost, vowed that he and Kennedy would take the battle to the Senate floor, where Nelson would propose the voluntary-mandatory approach and Kennedy would offer the mandatory program by itself, the administration's original proposal and the one the Human Resources Committee had, under Kennedy's guidance, approved in the summer of 1977.

The measure did not get brought before the Senate until a few days before adjournment for the election. Finally, on Thursday afternoon, October 12, the Senate took up the Talmadge bill. Kennedy offered his amendment first and after it was defeated by a 69–18 roll-call vote Nelson offered his voluntary-mandatory approach. Nelson's amendment, which supplemented the Medicare-Medicaid reforms being proposed by Talmadge, was finally accepted by a 47–42 roll-call vote. Then the entire bill was passed.[87]

Once the Senate passed the bill, the problem was how to get the measure before the House, which was already badly behind on its agenda and was still hoping to adjourn Saturday evening. Because the Senate-passed bill had a House bill number (a move that had been necessary to comport with congressional rules), the measure could theoretically go straight to conference.

House Speaker Tip O'Neill indicated that he was giving cost containment low priority. He had told the administration, he said, not to bother him about other legislation until the House completed work on the tax and energy bills. The general feeling was that the Senate has passed the measure expecting it to die in the House.

In fact, the day after the Senate passed the bill, Friday the 13th, during the daily leadership press conference on the floor of the Senate prior to starting the day's work, Ted Stevens, the assistant Republican leader, in response to a reporter's question as to why the Senate had adopted the Nelson amendment so easily, said, "The word was out that it would not go any place in the House and so senators could easily vote for it without concern."[88]

Nevertheless, the administration was eager to have the measure brought up in the House, and Ways and Means chief Al Ullman Friday noon convened his committee for the purpose of agreeing to accept the Senate version and bringing it back to the full House for an up-or-down vote. Lacking about four votes of the majority needed, the panel was unable to muster a quorum. At mid-afternoon on Friday, Califano, Ullman and Rostenkowski met in a back room off the House floor to plot further strategy. The agreed-upon plan provided that the administration would spearhead the mustering of the additional four votes needed, but try as they might advocates of the measure were unable to get the commitments from any more than seventeen of the nineteen Ways and Means Committee members needed to move the measure.

By late Saturday afternoon, even the administration had given up hope. One top HEW lobbyist said, "We can't make it. There's too little time and too much else on the agenda."[89] And Congress adjourned, bringing an end to the effort.

With Congress closed down, the hospital industry was able to argue that since that year's hospital inflation rate was more than two percentage points below the 15 percent-plus rate of earlier years, the voluntary effort was working and federal controls were not needed since hospitals by themselves could handle the task. Hospital spokesmen said that the industry had more than met its voluntary goal for 1978 and would be able to continue to gain control of health care inflation in 1979.

Alex McMahon, president of the American Hospital Association, said that the success of the voluntary effort was the "single most important factor in winning Congress' support in the fight against" the administration's program. The voluntary effort had saved $900 million in fiscal 1978, he said, and was expected to save an additional $4 billion through fiscal 1983.[90]

Later in the fall, Carter announced a new phase of his anti-inflation effort and once again he hammered away at the hospital industry:

> The health care industry is not one in which market forces can be expected to provide an adequate restraint on price increases. The most significant action we can take to reduce inflation in medical costs is to institute direct controls over hospital costs. Hospital costs are the largest and fastest growing component of medical care costs. They have increased between 15 and 20 percent in each of the last three years and now constitute 40 percent of total health care costs.[91]

Carter was determined not to let up on his effort to win enactment of his hospital cost-containment legislation; by then it had become an item in which he was taking a deeply personal interest.

Health Planning: A Burden Too Large

If the Carter administration could not immediately win enactment of its hospital cost-containment proposal, it could rely on legislation already on the books, the Health Planning Act, to help it try to hold down the rise in hospital costs, but it would be a weak reed on which to hold.

The 1974 Planning Act was the product of a recognition of a proliferation of federal health programs, often, it seemed, with little relation to one another, and of the substantial investment—some saw it as excessive—in hospital construction and equipment. The overinvestment resulted from several factors: the insurance system, hospitals competing for physicians by offering attractive equipment and facilities, and federal subsidies for hospital construction.

The new act, signed into law by President Ford on January 4, 1975, authorized spending $1 billion over a three-year period to subsidize the development of a national network of local and state health planning agencies and in other ways to improve planning for the use and development of health resources. The goal, besides bringing some rationality to health planning efforts, was to give states, communities and consumers a major say in how that planning would be carried out. But the program was also the product of other forces.

The Planning Act became law during the apex of the era when Congress and the Executive Branch were battling to achieve dominance in health policy-making. The country had just concluded the protracted experience of ousting from office a totally unsatisfactory president. Congress had passed the Budget Control and Impoundment Act as a device to give itself much greater authority in the budget-making process and to prevent the president from refusing to spend funds it wanted him to spend.

Furthermore, the Nixon years had been ones of inflation generally and particularly of health care costs that had been stopped only momentarily by Nixon's economic stabilization program, or wage and price freeze. The Health Planning Act was expected to assume a major role in the effort to control rising health care costs by bringing some order to a chaotic environment. And, like most programs directed at a specific problem, it was oversold—oversold by the administration that fostered it, oversold by its congressional sponsors, and oversold by the nongovernmental constituency that would develop the grass-roots support for its enactment. It was from the start expected to accomplish too much, and when, a few years later, it had not made much headway in achieving those goals, support for it diminished.

Legislation designed to build a health planning system was already on the books when work was begun on the 1974 law, but it had not been able to do the job. The Hill-Burton hospital construction program, first enacted in 1946, provided incentives for states to plan the development of health resources. Then legislation enacted during the Johnson Great Society years—the partnership for health, regional medical and comprehensive health planning programs—sought to strengthen the effort. But these programs were too narrowly focused and too much was happening during those years to permit them to do the job. A more comprehensive and sweeping program was needed—one that would implant a comprehensive planning system on the entire country and, while giving each community a good deal of discretion, would set the same standards for the entire nation.

Paul Rogers, the chairman of the House Commerce health subcommittee, saw the 1974 Planning Act as a logical development in the incremental process he so carefully fostered, and when his committee finally cleared the legislation he felt another major building block had been put in place. The report that his committee wrote said the new program built upon the experience of existing programs and sought "to combine their best features into one new health planning and resources development effort."[92]

Edward Kennedy, responsible for developing the legislation in the Senate, saw the new act in much the same light, but for him it also was a very important element in setting the stage for national health insurance. An important feature of Kennedy's NHI bill, the Health Security Act, heavily emphasized health planning and the development of the proper mix of health resources. As he opened hearings on the proposed legislation in March 1974, Kennedy said:

> I believe that a national health insurance plan will be implemented in the United States within a short period of time. It is absolutely essential that an effective mechanism for the identification and realization of identified goals as a matter of national health policy and a mechanism for the realization of those goals be complementary to such a health insurance program.[93]

The pending legislation was designed, he said, to correct the deficiencies in existing legislation and to help develop the foundation for national health insurance.

The program as enacted in 1974, just after the Nixon-congressional clash had been resolved by Nixon's resignation, was very detailed. It had ten national priorities for planning the nation's health care system, everything from ensuring that the poor had adequate health care services, developing new systems of care such as health maintenance organizations, ensuring enough medical care personnel, building better prevention programs, and ensuring quality health care: the burden was heavy. The act spelled out also, in some detail, how its various provisions should be carried out; in this way it dramatically reflected the feeling in Congress that the Executive Branch, regardless of who sat in the White House, could not be entrusted to carry out on its own initiative broadly defined congressional intentions.

The mainstay of the program was the health systems agency, of which there would ultimately be two hundred in various communities throughout the country. These groups were to be governed by local residents, a majority of whom would be laypeople representing the community generally and the rest providers of health care services, such as physicians and nurses or hospital administrators.

Although the program became law in January 1975, like so many health programs it got off to a slow start. In fact, it was Joe Califano's HEW in the fall of 1977 that issued the first guidelines for the program, almost three years after the law had been enacted. Those guidelines, designed to complement the hospital cost-containment legislation that only a few months earlier had been put before Congress, reflected Califano's strong regulatory bias by seeking to check the rise in hospital costs through controlling the number of hospital beds and other hospital services.

The principal device in the Health Planning Act for controlling costs was called the certificate-of-need, a procedure under which planning agencies had to give permission, after a certain level of expenditure was involved, for the construction of a new facility, expansion of an existing one, or for the purchase of expensive, high-technology equipment if used in a hospital.

Of all the provisions of the Planning Act, it was the certificate-of-need (CON) provision that proved to be the most controversial, for it was a truly regulatory provision that held the potential for ultimate total federal control over the health care marketplace. CON was the device that was to hold down excessive investment in health care facilities. Before a new hospital could be constructed, an existing one expanded, or before a hospital could purchase an expensive piece of equipment, the state health planning agency had to give its concurrence in this need by granting a certificate, a CON. Approval to purchase equipment went directly to the heart of the hospitals' ability to attract patients, for to attract patients they needed to attract doctors. To do that they must offer equipment and facilities at least as advanced, technologically, as other hospitals in the area.

A principal target of CON, at least at first, was the scanner, first designed to view the brain and later the entire body. Affectionately called the CAT or CT scanner, for computerized axial tomography, it combined techniques of X ray with computer technology to give cross-sectional views of the body's interior. The CAT sees not only the bones, but the soft tissues as well.

The CAT scanner was viewed with considerable jaundice by health planners because of its potential for raising the magnitude of health care costs. But most medical practitioners saw the scanner as a device that had transformed the diagnosis and treatment of the brain, as well as other parts of the body. A 1981 conference on CAT scanners sponsored by the National Institutes of Health concluded that there were too few, not too many, scanners. Indeed, many viewed the CAT scanner as being just as valuable a piece of medical equipment as the X ray. It was not so much that there were too many CAT scanners, but that they were poorly distributed.

Even though the certificate-of-need system sought to put a check on scanners, there were in 1981 about 1,300 scanners in the United States, one-third of the total number in the world. Although the first scans were introduced about 1972, the ones in use by the 1980s were several generations beyond the original models; in fact, the first models were then largely part of medical history and largely in museums.

The cost of purchasing scanners was not insignificant, and the industry that produced them was large. Prices ranged between $100,000 and $1 million, depending on the instrument's complexity. Likewise, the cost of using a scanner could be high—between $200 and $300 for each patient scan. The 1981 NIH conference concluded, however, that scans had actually helped decrease medical costs. Instead of more lengthy and complicated procedures, which might require hospitalization and exploratory surgery, the scan could produce the desired information in much less time, with much less agony and perhaps less cost. Scans, for example, replaced procedures for the diagnosis of pituitary tumors that before cost as much as $3,000. In 1982, the world market for CAT scanners reached $730 million, and in the five-year period ending in 1987, 1,100 hospitals in the United States were expected to purchase their first scanner and an additional 800 would purchase replacement units. Another 175 hospitals would expand existing units.[94]

But despite its value, many people, largely because of its cost, viewed the CAT scan with considerable reservation. By some estimates, at least half of all scans were not necessary, and each such procedure raised not only the cost of the patient's care but also exposed him to radiation. Furthermore, if the scan revealed the need for surgery, the physicians at the hospital giving the scan might decide to do it, although that hospital and those physicians might not be the appropriate ones, the most skilled, for the job. As the surplus of doctors pressed more fiercely on the large urban and academic centers where physicians traditionally congregated and where the more elaborate medical care was carried out, more doctors moved to small communities and rural areas. As that happened, there was more pressure on the small, community hospitals where they practiced to purchase CAT scanners, and thus an even greater likelihood that, based on the diagnosis produced by the scan, surgery would be performed there, perhaps inappropriately.

Containing costs, however, was not the only job of the health planning program. It was also expected to help redress what many considered the fundamental problem of the nation's health care system—the lack of market competition. When the Planning Act was renewed in 1979, this task was emphasized. By the time the legislation was considered, the debate over competition in the health care sector was in full swing. David Stockman, at that time a Republican representative from Michigan on the Commerce health subcommittee and later Reagan's budget director, was a strong advocate of reducing government regulation that he argued hurt competition. He did not accept the argument that medical costs were being driven up because hospitals were buying too many CAT scanners and other high-technology equipment. High-quality health care was going to cost more, and there was no way to prevent that, he argued. If the federal government clamped down on such a trend, he maintained, it would chill the climate for innovation in medical technology and treatment. The planning program in general and the certificates-of-need in particular would lead to a public utility-type regulation if allowed to go the full course. This would limit entry into the market of new products, and the result would be higher costs and lower quality. Those already in the market would become entrenched and dominate it. The solution, Stockman suggested, was to ask providers and consumers to develop a higher regard for the costs of the services they were demanding.

The Health Planning Act was renewed in 1979, and the most striking new feature of this new act was its emphasis on the need for the health planning system to stimulate traditional marketplace competition in the health services industry. Although both the House and Senate bills contained similar language as the measures emerged from committee, it was in the House that the most extensive debate on the possibilities of free enterprise in the health care system took place. The debate was the beginning of one that would permeate consideration of health issues for years to come.

The 1979 legislation extended the planning program for three years, but it was to be downhill from then on. The Reagan administration, with Stockman in a central role to dictate health policy, viewed health planning as unnecessary government intervention, and although the program survived the first two years of Reagan's term, its support was waning. The competition debate would then be carried on separately.

NHI—Carter's First Round

It was generally assumed when Senator Edward Kennedy took on President Jimmy Carter at the midterm Democratic convention in Memphis, in December 1978, where he strongly criticized the president on a number of domestic issues, including his health program, that he was starting a campaign for the presidency. Kennedy, indeed, may already, in his own mind, have decided to run for the Democratic Party's nomination, but that did not have to be the case in order to explain his attack on Carter's program.

Even though he was a Kennedy, in pursuing his legislative goals in the Senate Edward Kennedy had to compete for attention with lots of other folk. He was firmly dedicated to his goal of a national health insurance program and wanted very much for it to materialize. One way to make sure his idea was given respectful attention throughout the land was to let it be reported in the context of his ambitions for the presidency. There is no question that the prospect for NHI moved along more rapidly than it otherwise might have because the issue was presented within this framework. Ironically, it is also a major reason why no national health insurance program has been enacted, for the issue got caught up in the riptide of presidential ambitions.

Long before Carter was viewed as a presidential contender, even perhaps before he seriously thought of himself in that role, Kennedy had been in the candidate's ring, and he knew how to play the game well.

Although Kennedy's personal ideology firmly supported the concept embedded in the Health Security Act, his political pragmatism led him to abandon it at times. He first cast the original plan aside, as noted earlier, in 1974 to join with Wilbur Mills, who was then chairman of the House Ways and Means Committee, in sponsoring a hybrid version that they thought might make some headway at a time when Mills was pursuing his ambitions for higher office.

It did not succeed, and Kennedy returned to the Health Security Act, primarily as a staging area from which to move out again on national health insurance at a later time; he knew he would have to move away from the Health Security Act the next time NHI moved forward, but in keeping with his practice of setting a goal beyond that which could realistically be attained he returned to the original proposal.

Although he had gotten more recognition than any other member of Congress for his advocacy of national health insurance, Kennedy was actually a minor player in the initial congressional activity over NHI. In the House, jurisdiction over the proposal was split between the Commerce and Ways and Means Committees, but in the Senate jurisdiction lay almost exclusively with the Finance Committee. Although Kennedy as chairman of the Human Resources health subcommittee held hearings on the issue and NHI legislation was jointly referred to his committee, the dominant role in drafting the program, nevertheless, lay with the Finance Committee. It would not be until a bill actually came to the Senate floor that Kennedy would have an adequate shot at imposing his views on national health insurance legislation, but by then much of the preliminary work would be done and it might be too late. That was one important reason why Kennedy wanted President Carter to adopt his, Kennedy's, proposal and push it as his own.

For the first year of Carter's administration, national health insurance remained essentially a dormant issue, with the White House timetable for publishing the president's plan constantly slipping—slippages that went largely unnoticed. The new administration during this year was gearing up on all fronts, and in the health area it was focusing on hospital cost containment.

Skeptics argued that the slippage was intentional, that Carter never wanted a national health insurance program enacted during his first term. The skeptics claimed that activity over NHI during the Carter years was a charade, and that there was no serious, substantive pursuit of NHI in the latter part of the 1970s. In the memoirs of his presidency, Carter gave very little attention to domestic issues, except the energy problem, and health issues—primarily national health insurance and hospital cost containment—got only a few pages, thus in some ways corroborating the skeptics' view. Carter in fact probably was leery of the possible adverse political impact of national health insurance should its expectations not materialize—certainly he was wary of its cost—but the public record is unequivocal: Carter presented a plan, he asked that it be enacted, and he and his emissaries at the time aggressively pursued that objective. There is no dispute, though, that Carter did want to delay spending under a national health insurance program, should one be enacted, as long as possible.

The first word from the new president was that his plan would be ready to go to Congress in the fall of 1977.

But work did not proceed as fast as he originally planned. A major obstacle was the need for considerable thought about the overwhelming task of implementing a national health insurance program once it was enacted and the serious apprehension that its costs would become so great that they would hang as an albatross around the neck of an administration firmly committed to holding down federal spending. Another was the desire to minimize as much as possible friction with Carter's supporters outside the administration. But some of that friction was generated from within. Joe Califano sought to dominate the shaping of Carter's national health insurance proposal.

The Carter administration during its early days was designed to be a cabinet-run government. Cabinet officers were given considerable flexibility about how to pursue their responsibilities for developing policy and new programs. Later, the responsibility was somewhat recentralized in the White House, but during the first year or so, the opportunity for initiative lay primarily with the departments. And Califano was one to exploit that prerogative to the fullest. But there were limitations even within this framework.

Carter had said early in his administration that he wanted reform of the nation's welfare programs given top priority. This task fell to Califano, just as development of a national health insurance plan had, and although in a conceptual sense the two were closely related, they were both very large tasks and would require a great deal of effort. They were conceptually related because the existing federal health program for the poor, Medicaid, was linked in terms of who was eligible for care, to eligibility for welfare.

Nevertheless, there were some in the young Carter administration—such as Stuart Eizenstat, the president's chief of domestic programs, and Peter Bourne, a special advisor on mental health and related issues—who thought national health insurance and hospital cost containment should move along in tandem—one could not be successful without the other, and thus they argued that national health insurance should be made ready to go forward with hospital cost containment before the administration's first spring passed.[95]

But Califano was not ready to move so fast, and he first established an advisory committee to help educate the new leaders in the department on national health insurance issues. Then he set about developing a set of option papers that looked at national health insurance from different angles.

If Califano was proceeding at his own pace, he nevertheless believed that Carter was not sufficiently focused on the national health insurance issue and did not really want to have to deal with the matter at that point. In May 1977 Califano met with Kennedy at the latter's home to talk about NHI and he told Kennedy he should push Carter on the subject—bring public pressure on the president to move more rapidly.[96]

Kennedy did just that. Shortly thereafter both he and the president were scheduled to speak to the annual convention of the United Auto Workers in Los Angeles, with Kennedy speaking first. It was the last convention for Leonard Woodcock, who was retiring, and the event was mainly one to laud the outgoing president. Kennedy did that, but he also launched into a need for more rapid progress on national health insurance. Carter followed Kennedy the next day, and changed his prepared text to emphasize his desire to move forward rapidly on NHI.

But it was not until that November that Carter himself got his first briefing on national health insurance, and then he said the plan would come forward in early 1978. One of the main issues to come up at the

November briefing was the prospect of organized labor criticizing Carter for backing away from the Kennedy Health Security Act if Carter proposed a plan using insurance companies. Carter reportedly said at that meeting, "Labor is wrong. I was the only Democratic candidate who did not endorse the Kennedy bill during the campaign."[97]

One of Califano's first steps in developing an NHI plan was to contract with a former colleague with whom he had worked in the Defense Department in the early days of John Kennedy's administration. Alain Enthoven, like Califano, had been one of Robert McNamara's whiz kids at the Pentagon. Now he was a professor at Stanford University, and Califano called on him to develop a national health insurance proposal for the new administration. What Enthoven delivered to Califano in the fall of 1977 was a hybrid device that took off from the existing concepts used to provide health insurance to federal employees and it went on from there to rely heavily on the prepaid concept embedded in the health maintenance organization and to emphasize the need for more competition in the health care field.

Enthoven's plan was sympathetically received in the White House, but it was soon rejected when it became clear that it strayed so far from the Kennedy-labor concept of what a national health insurance program should be like that it would never be accepted by that group. What is more, the event had more serious consequences. This was the first round for the Carter administration in developing a national health insurance plan, and the document was a clear signal to Kennedy and labor that Califano, who they had expected because of his liberal credentials and background would be squarely in their camp, let alone Carter, was not going to accept the Health Security Act lock, stock and barrel.

Califano sent four different proposals to the president in early 1978. One was Enthoven's plan to restore traditional competition to the health care marketplace. The second focused on comprehensive care for the poor and catastrophic health insurance for everyone, following the approach used by Senators Russell Long and Abraham Ribicoff. The third required employers to provide health insurance for all employees and also proposed a public plan for those not employed. The fourth was patterned after Kennedy's Health Security Act—an entirely public plan with strong federal controls over how much could be spent.

As soon as Califano began to deviate from specifics that had been laid down by Carter in his Student National Medical Association speech, and that now were so jealously coveted by organized labor in general and the United Auto Workers in particular, he ran into trouble.

Hamilton Jordan and other political advisors in the White House were, at least in the early days of the Carter administration, very concerned about remaining in the good graces of organized labor. As Califano deviated from the original concepts and as the word got out, the UAW would immediately get in touch with Jordan to voice its concerns. This was part of the reason for such intense frustration within this White House group with Califano, for he was not respecting the political bond that had been created during the campaign. When Jordan would then try to get Califano in line, he would be unsuccessful.

Califano saw his role, in part, as that of broker between Carter and Kennedy. He was well aware of the enmity Carter felt for Kennedy and of his fear that the Massachusetts senator would oppose him in 1980. Califano knew that if the Carter administration was to have a successful national health insurance plan it would have to meet with Kennedy's approval, but he also knew that he was going to have to develop a plan that would not cost as much as the Kennedy plan if he was going to get the support of other administration officials and important members of the House, like Al Ullman.[98]

Kennedy met with Carter in December 1977 to discuss national health insurance. He wanted to work out a compromise, Kennedy said. Carter was frank about what he wanted—to involve the insurance companies, keep the costs down, and have as much of the money as possible flow through the private sector, which meant requiring employers to purchase health insurance for their employees. Kennedy, in response, set up a work group headed by Larry Horowitz, a physician who was his principal aide on health issues and staff director of his health subcommittee, and this group set about writing a new Kennedy national health insurance plan that would meet the president's stipulations. Unlike 1974, when Kennedy deviated from the Health Security Act, the UAW, this time, was heavily involved in writing the new proposal.[99]

By March, Horowitz's group had completed writing a draft that responded to Carter's requirements, and Kennedy and Douglas Fraser, the new UAW president, had agreed to it. Horowitz brought it to Stuart Eizenstat, who found much in it that the White House could agree with. But Califano's work at HEW was also moving along. The four plans had already been submitted to the president. There now was a lot on the table.

When 1978 dawned, most expected that the administration would make public its NHI principles before many weeks passed. But national health insurance was significantly downplayed in both the budget and the State of the Union messages that went to Congress early in the year, and delays defeated the expectation that an announcement was imminent. The administration wasn't yet ready.

Kennedy's willingness to back off, and organized labor, reluctantly, with him, from his previously tightly held position that NHI should be a totally federally financed and run program, was a substantial concession from the senator. Carter and Kennedy appeared headed toward a compromise that would leave the principal role with private insurance companies but subject them to a system of federal charter and regulation. The two met in April, and it was publicly reported that they had reached "broad agreement." Carter's principles on national health insurance, which would be endorsed by Kennedy, would be made public by summer, and the legislation would go to Congress by fall. This was a compromise that would never be consummated, and it set the pattern for repeated near misses in compromises between Kennedy and Carter.

The spring meeting had the seeds of the strife to follow. Labor leaders also were present at the meeting with Carter on April 6, 1978. Kennedy told Carter of his work on a new plan that would involve insurance companies, as Carter wanted. But Kennedy also told the president that he and labor would stand firm on the "principles of universality, comprehensive benefits and tough controls." He and labor, he added, were looking toward national health insurance as an issue in the fall's congressional elections. Califano in his memoirs described the meeting as one in which Kennedy was saying things for the benefit of the leaders of organized labor who were present at the meeting. He said that Kennedy was "almost disdainful" of Carter and that he pressed Carter on the procedure that would be used to develop the plan. He wanted to be an intimate part of that process. Carter reminded Kennedy that during the campaign he had not supported the Health Security Act but instead "endorsed a set of principles."[100]

Six weeks later, on May 19, Carter met with Senators Russell Long, Herman Talmadge and Abraham Ribicoff, who warned the president against adopting the Kennedy plan. They argued for their proposal that federalized Medicaid and established a program of catastrophic health insurance. Long maintained that the Kennedy plan, which he said was what was meant by Carter's principles, was simply an effort by the UAW to get health off the bargaining table by having the federal government pay for the cost of all health care.[101]

In the meantime, Carter was also getting strong counsel from his economic advisors that national health insurance, at least a plan that cost the federal government any substantial amount of new money, would seriously undermine his economic plan. Michael Blumenthal, secretary of the Treasury, and James McIntyre, director of the Office of Management and Budget, along with Charles Schultze, chairman of the Council of Economic Advisors, were unanimously opposed to expensive new domestic programs. They saw mounting budget deficits and an economy that was contracting, not expanding, and they believed a national health insurance program that required substantial federal investment would be self-defeating. Even if it were enacted, which they doubted (they did not believe the support was there in Congress), the money necessary to finance it could not be raised without causing substantial stress on the federal budget. New dollars were no longer available to the federal government as they had been in the 1960s and early 1970s when the economy had been expanding. The economic posture of the United States had changed, and it was not just a matter of wading through a trough. The change was long term.

The most that Schultze and the other presidential economic advisors would go along with was a catastrophic health insurance plan, and perhaps improvements in Medicaid to help the poor.

What is more, a national health insurance program, at least along the lines of Kennedy's Health Security Act, would simply substitute public dollars for private ones. It made no sense, Schultze believed, to put the economy through such a wrenching experience—changing the path along which these health dollars flowed—to accomplish little change, except perhaps to have the federal government gain control over who was paid how much.

The liberalism of the Kennedy and Johnson years, when Schultze had served as director of the Bureau of the Budget, the predecessor to the Office of Management and Budget, was no longer feasible. Now the government, Schultze believed, was in a transition from expansion to a posture of restraint. The economy was no longer performing as well as it had into the early years of the Nixon administration, and this made it doubly difficult to expand the concepts of responsibilities of a welfare society.[102]

The rhetoric used by both Carter and Kennedy to describe their differences over NHI, although appearing trivial, was important because, as in all politically sensitive matters of this sort, the framework in which the issue moves forward is more important than the substance of the proposal. Carter made it clear that he wanted a consensus bill, and to achieve that he apparently believed at first that he needed the support not only of Kennedy and the labor coalition that had been the prime citizen support for the senator's Health Security Act, but also of the health insurance industry as well as other members of Congress.

In addition to saying that national health insurance must have a role for the insurance industry, Carter insisted that its impact on the federal budget must be minimal. The two presidential requirements for NHI meant that the administration's proposal would ensure the continuation of the underwriting role for the insurance companies, which in turn meant that the companies would be allowed to make a profit. In exchange for an agreement to accept this approach, Kennedy and labor in the spring of 1978 were demanding a commitment from the administration that it would propose regulating the insurance industry in a way that would put a limit on those profits. They were also insisting that coverage be comprehensive and uniform, that barriers to health care such as deductibles and coinsurance be virtually eliminated, that the program emphasize outpatient rather than hospital care, and that prospective budgeting or setting annual limits by geographic area on how much could be spent for different types of health services must be an integral part of the scheme. Many, but not all, of these principles were ones to which Carter had committed himself during the 1976 campaign.

By the time of the Carter-Kennedy negotiations in the spring of 1978, however, there was a deep schism between the White House staff and

HEW over how the plan should be developed and written. Those responsible for national health insurance issues in each place were becoming increasingly suspicious of their counterparts. The White House staff, particularly the political advisors, believed that Califano and his troops were trying to go too far in accommodating Kennedy, and Kennedy's softened stand in April only reinforced that suspicion.

The White House staff, and the president himself, were persuaded by the argument of economic advisors to proceed with a limited catastrophic plan. Such a plan would have not only a minimum impact on the budget—perhaps as little as $5 billion a year, depending on how it was written—but would probably also have the best chance in Congress, where many leaders, particularly in the House, were leery of national health insurance because of the potential cost, and because the catastrophic approach was that favored by Russell Long.

Hamilton Jordan continued to be primarily concerned about the political consequences of Carter's national health insurance decision on organized labor and particularly on the United Auto Workers. At a meeting with economic and political advisors on March 2, 1978, Carter was starting to move away from his 1976 statements. Jordan stepped in to try to counteract it. "The president has a political commitment to the UAW," Jordan said. "At a time where our public opinion polls are down," he added, "we've got to stay close to powerful organizations like this." Carter replied, "My word is at stake. I have made a commitment."[103] But what he saw as his commitment was to release principles in 1978, not a full bill. During this period, Califano found House leaders—Ullman and Rostenkowski—cool to the idea of a national health insurance proposal. They did not even want principles released, let alone a bill. All members of the House in November would face reelection from constituents who were becoming increasingly concerned about the cost of government, and some, like those in California who had voted for Proposition 13, were forcing their state governments to reduce their tax burden.

But Califano and HEW were proceeding to push a broader plan. Much more than the White House, with the economic advisors now dominating opinion, they wanted a program that would provide not only more benefits and more coverage but that would also attempt to reform the nation's health care system. The plan that Califano finally submitted was not what the White House believed it had asked for, and the staff there saw too much of Kennedy in it. The Califano plan helped to confirm the belief held by the president's political advisors, primarily Hamilton Jordan, that the HEW secretary was more a Kennedy booster than a Carter advocate. If such a plan were adopted by the president and if it were enacted, Kennedy would get the credit, and that was unthinkable. Jordan now started backing away from the bond with the United Auto Workers that he had so assiduously nurtured a few months earlier.

What is more, the White House staff in 1978 was becoming increasingly concerned about rising inflation and the vanishing prospects of a balanced budget, one of the reasons for the continued focus on hospital cost containment. Because of inflation and because Congress could not be persuaded to enact a fully comprehensive plan, it decided, therefore, that it would be better to back off from Carter's 1976 campaign statements about national health insurance.

By early June 1978, Carter was wavering from his commitment to the principles of comprehensiveness. In a meeting with his advisors he said it would be "ridiculous to think about endorsing a bill like Kennedy's. I am not going to destroy my credibility on inflation and budgetary matters. I intend to be honest and responsible with the American people."[104] But exactly how to proceed had yet to be decided—whether to go for a Long-type targeted plan of catastrophic health insurance or for a more comprehensive one that would cover more people.

The climax came in July. Carter and Kennedy broke—irrevocably it turned out, although there were efforts to mend the break—over national health insurance, and the break was preceded by a series of political flurries that had the flavor of a summit conference. During the last week of July Carter tried to get Kennedy to join with him to support the principles he was about to release, principles that differed little in substance from those he had stipulated as a candidate. Kennedy of course had lauded those, but now he would say they were inadequate. Carter's announcement was put off several times in the hope of reaching an accommodation with Kennedy.

Carter and Kennedy met alone on Wednesday, July 26, 1978, at 5:00 P.M., and afterward Carter was still optimistic about an accommodation.

Califano, the broker, continued to meet with Kennedy, and by July 27, he says, he had come to an agreement, on all but two issues—a commitment to a single bill and a fixed schedule for phasing-in the program. If it had to be changed, Kennedy, according to Califano, wanted Congress to change the law; he did not want to have the administration able to change the plan unilaterally. Kennedy believed that more than one bill would allow Long and his Finance Committee to take the issue away from him.[105] But the issues were deeper than that. Kennedy felt very strongly that there had to be a commitment to a full, comprehensive plan from the beginning and that plan had to be embedded in legislation, which would be enacted. That way, the United States government, regardless of who sat in the White House or which party controlled Congress, would be fully committed to a comprehensive and universal national health insurance program. If it were to be altered subsequently, the whole legislative process would have to be run again when he and his allies would have a solid chance of keeping their gains. If the phase-in schedule was not a solid commitment, then the president, Carter or someone else, could unilaterally curtail the plan. Some argued that the phase-in issue was trivial, that Kennedy could leap that hurdle just as he had leapt others—particularly the issue of the role of insurance companies.

But Kennedy did not view it as trivial—it was to him very important and very substantial. He had indeed made large concessions to Carter, the magnitude of which he felt Carter did not fully appreciate, and he was having his own problems with advisors. Unlike 1974, in 1978 Kennedy did not leave the labor-citizen coalition when he started negotiating a new NHI plan with the president. This group was involved in the effort from the beginning, and while they came along, some came along very reluctantly.

Max Fine, the director of the Health Security Action Council, wanted to develop a solid compromise, one that would give national health insurance a foot in the door of the legislative process, and he knew Kennedy well enough to believe that Kennedy would compromise further as the legislative process got underway—he would have to; that was what enacting legislation was all about. Fine expected that Kennedy would later on drop his insistence on no deductibles and coinsurance. But the objective now was to get Kennedy and Carter to agree on a workable compromise so that union was forged.[106]

Stuart Eizenstat, during those days in late July, was working along with Kennedy, too, primarily with Kennedy's aide Larry Horowitz, and both felt, each reported later in interviews, that had they been allowed to work out a compromise without the additional political forces bearing in on them, they would have been successful—but that compromise, they both made clear four years later, would have had to involve Carter's making a solid commitment regarding phasing-in.

By early summer of 1978, not only was Carter's economic team against commitments for a phase-in, but Hamilton Jordan and Carter's other political advisors were now against making an alliance with Kennedy. They were convinced by that time that Kennedy would run against Carter—they did not believe him when he said he would not—and they were beginning to feel that they had lost the support of the UAW; perhaps seeking the union's continued support was no longer worth the payment required. Meanwhile, Califano was also pushing a compromise plan—one that involved a commitment to a phased-in schedule of benefits—and this exasperated the White House political staff even more.

The feeling that Kennedy would run against Carter in 1980 provided the momentum toward a self-fulfilling prophecy.

Carter and Kennedy held one last meeting on Friday morning, July 28. At that meeting, Carter was reportedly rough, stating his desires and what he could do; Kennedy argued again for a single bill. "If it is not one bill, then your words have little meaning—especially when phasing is based on forces we have very little control over. That is the heart of the issue." He said he would lose his constituency if there was more than one bill. Kennedy said Carter could not get his bill through Congress. After the meeting, Kennedy called Califano and asked again for a compromise (i.e., for Carter to accept his demands). He said he was being hounded by the press for comment and would have to respond to the issue publicly that afternoon unless they were able to agree to a compromise. Califano said that the announcement would not be made until Saturday morning, July 29, but Kennedy wanted the announcement that afternoon—he couldn't wait.[107]

For Carter to shield himself from the press was easy, and it was relatively easy for his staff and cabinet officers who had sufficient institutional trappings to give them privacy when they wanted it. But it was not so easy for Kennedy who had to move about in the corridors of the Capitol and the Senate office buildings to do his job and who had no private escapes or elevators to take him from his office. Besides, Kennedy liked the press and often enjoyed meetings with them. He felt, and his staff did too, that he could not avoid the press stake-out, including a full array of television cameras, until Califano—who told Kennedy that his charts were not yet ready; that's why he could not move that afternoon—held his news conference scheduled for Saturday morning.

But other forces were at work on Kennedy. There was already talk that he was planning to run for the Democratic presidential nomination against Carter in 1980, and clearly some people, primarily those around him, had a stake in his doing so. It was impossible for them to consider the events of the moment outside of the larger context of the possible 1980 race. If Kennedy upstaged Carter on national health insurance and did it in a way that had credibility, it would help Kennedy lay the groundwork for a 1980 race.

Now, national health insurance, which had moved so far through the political process precisely because Kennedy was viewed as a potential presidential candidate, was running aground because he was considering fulfilling that expectation.

While there were still substantive differences between Kennedy and Carter over the ingredients of an NHI plan, by this time they were minimal when compared to the gulf that had stood between them at the time of the 1976 election and even more so when the whole history of the national health insurance effort was drawn into the picture.

Kennedy was more willing to compromise on the substance of his program than on its politics. He argued that while the program could be implemented over a period of years, it must be enacted as one package. He felt that this was necessary in order to keep the support of both organized labor and the citizens' coalition that was providing the grassroots support. The citizens' coalition, however, probably would have followed Kennedy along any path he chose, for they were dedicated to him and besides had no place else to go. As a practical matter, labor would probably have chosen to follow Kennedy's lead as well had he chosen to make further accommodations with Carter, for it, too, had no place to go except to Carter, which perhaps was what worried Kennedy.

If Kennedy were to fully accommodate Carter, the difference between the two in a 1980 primary and convention fight, at least over health issues, would be muted and Kennedy would lose that leverage over labor.

Organized labor by the summer of 1978 was frustrated and annoyed with Carter, and Kennedy, sensing that feeling, was making it possible for himself to fill the gap. He recalled too vividly 1974, when he had lost labor's support by developing a compromise bill with Wilbur Mills, and Kennedy did not want to get caught in that predicament again. He also recalled labor's strong commitment to Carter in 1976 and perhaps speculated that it was best to drive in the wedge as soon as he could.

Much of the problem in developing an NHI plan during the Carter administration had to do with personalities, and each one came out tarnished. Joe Califano, like Kennedy, came from the liberal Democratic mold, but, unlike Kennedy, had great difficulty working as a team player; he tended to go off on his own. It was a difficult relationship for Kennedy; there was strain, and the strain reached down to their staffs. It became increasingly difficult for all people to work together.

Kennedy even brought this to Carter's attention, and although Carter by this time was becoming increasingly disillusioned with Califano, there was nothing he could do to rein in the secretary. Califano would do things unilaterally and then expect the administration's natural allies in Congress to accept them afterward.

But Carter, too, was difficult to deal with, and erratic. In that last week before the final break with Kennedy, Carter had let things get out of control. Stuart Eizenstat, chief of Carter's domestic council staff, on Thursday, July 27, had told Jim Corman, the principal House cosponsor of Kennedy's Health Security Act who would ultimately switch to the Carter plan, that the principles would not be released for another ten days. Kennedy for his part was not fully in control of his own agenda. The forces within his camp were pushing him toward a public and dramatic break with Carter, one that would make it even more difficult to mend the differences later on.[108]

Kennedy thus decided to make his break with Carter public, and he did so on Friday afternoon, July 28, in a press conference jointly held with AFL-CIO president George Meany and other labor leaders. He broke with the president, Kennedy said, because Carter would not make a commitment to send a single NHI bill to Congress or provide assurance that his program would move forward on a specific schedule regardless of national economic conditions. He said he had believed Carter had agreed with him on the "need for a program that would be universal in its application to all Americans, and comprehensive in the health benefits that would be covered," but, he added, there had been "two areas that go to the heart of the issue and the program" where he and Carter were not able to come to agreement. Kennedy wanted a "commitment to a single bill that would enable Congress to deal with the program as a whole, rather than allow it to be divided into separate bills and conquered by special interest groups . . . [and] a commitment that the proposal would not contain any built-in self destruct buttons," such as curtailing the plan if inflation rose too high. Carter's failure to make these two commitments, Kennedy said, cast doubt on his "commitment to a program that is universal and comprehensive—they draw into question whether in fact all Americans will finally be covered by the program, and whether in fact the benefits that are available will be comprehensive."

Carter's principles were a step in the right direction, Kennedy said, "but they are unacceptable overall, in light of our failure to reach agreement on the two important areas of our concern."

Kennedy said he hoped that the current break with the White House could be repaired, but in the meantime he and his labor colleagues intended to proceed on their own, "with the administration if possible, without the administration if necessary," to develop an NHI program. Kennedy concluded his opening remarks to the press by saying that he would continue to support the president on other issues in the future, adding, "But on this central and critical issue of health care in America, I regret to say that I believe the president has misread the mood of the people in this country and the strong support that exists for national health insurance . . . The president's failure of leadership on this issue now will make our effort more difficult in the future. But we shall work harder, and I am confident we shall prevail."[109]

But some of what Kennedy had to say was political jousting. The substantial issues, while still evident, were now seriously muted. Kennedy did not here or later criticize Carter for proposing a two-class system of care because financing of health care for the poor would be different than that for the rest of the population. Nor did he criticize Carter for not proposing a national health care budget, an idea that was crucial in Kennedy's view to containing inflation in health care costs. These distinctions were a critical weakness in the Kennedy national health insurance lexicon, and Kennedy's failure to point to them at the press conference seemed to reveal his purpose as being more political than ideological.

Kennedy and labor argued that without a firm plan with a firm schedule set forth in a single piece of legislation the consumer would be asked to pay the consequences when federal budgetary control faltered, costs in the health care industry continued to rise, or some other arbitrary event prevented the triggering of the next phase of the national health insurance plan.

Kennedy said he, labor and the citizens' coalition supporting the Health Security Act would set to work writing a new bill that would be responsive to the concerns expressed by the administration but that would also provide for universal and comprehensive coverage with assurance that different phases would be implemented according to a specified schedule.

Kennedy's concerns, however, as noted, can be viewed in the last analysis only as a device for breaking with Carter. Kennedy had gone a long way toward compromising with Carter and he could easily have gone the rest of the way; when the final moment came, however, he chose not to, and by doing so put national health insurance in peril. But in Kennedy's view, entering into a pact with Carter after having compromised his own position so substantially involved some serious risks, for Carter had proven, from Kennedy's point of view, to be extremely quixotic—Carter might back off further once a pact had been made; he could not be trusted.

Four years later, through interviews, there would be a difference in opinion by Kennedy allies as to why Kennedy could not accept Carter's plan. The reasons stated by Kennedy—the failure to agree to a single bill and that the elements of the plan would be phased-in as scheduled regardless of economic conditions—were not the whole story.

A fundamental difference between the Carter and Kennedy plans as they finally emerged was the kind of health insurance program—and thus the kind of care—to which different groups of people would have access. Under the Kennedy approach, everyone, regardless of income level or location, would have access, through insurance, to all providers, and thus there would be only one level, in theory, of quality of care. Under Carter's plan there would be two systems. The employed and well-to-do would have their health care paid for through the traditional health insurance system where there would be much fewer controls over providers, while the poor, near-poor, and others such as the elderly who used the public plan, would get their health insurance through a federally subsidized and run program that would control physician fees and hospital rates. The danger would be that those using the public plan ran the risk of getting less careful attention from the health care system because the payment for their services would not be as good.

The issue of the one-class system of health care is an important one in the liberal Democratic Party ethic, for it is another step in eliminating the differences between people with different income levels. But this was not the point Kennedy emphasized when criticizing Carter's plan, and later it was the objection to Carter's plan cited by only some of his supporters. Others argued that the essential difference lay in the ability of the Kennedy plan to reform the health care system, and in the Carter plan's inability to do so. Carter's plan would simply continue the existing fee-for-service system, even though some limits would be put on part of it, Kennedy's allies would argue, while Kennedy's plan would establish a budgeting system that would set in advance each year how much each provider could spend—a prospective budgeting system that would require providers to live within a predetermined spending plan. The trouble with such plans, however, was that when the final arbitraor is the federal government, the budget can be breached and often quite easily so, through the political process; it would be a partial barrier to excessive inflation in health care costs, not a total one.

Although organized labor and particularly the UAW criticized the new Carter plan as inadequate, had it been enacted it would have relieved labor of one of its most severe problems, just as the Kennedy plan would have. It would help in contract negotiations. Initially, the incorporation of health insurance costs into the fringe-benefits package negotiated by labor had been a big plus, for it meant in practical terms more income for the workers without that income being taxed, and this initially was advantageous to management because it meant that they would not have to pay social security taxes on these wages. But by the end of the 1970s, the cost of health benefits had become huge for management—especially for the automobile companies, where they added several hundred dollars to the cost of each car. Managements were beginning to resist this fringe benefit as their own profits were disappearing. Thus, to labor there was some advantage in getting the cost of health care off the bargaining table, and the only way to do that was achieve enactment of national health insurance that would be paid for entirely by the federal government, or which mandated that employers purchase a certain level of care for their employees. This the Carter plan would do, although, as under any type of plan, contract negotiations could take up the issue of supplementary insurance.

Even though Kennedy was a traditional Democratic liberal who was used to doing things in the incremental way, he had come to believe that in the health arena the incremental approach would only exacerbate the problem and in the long run cause the system to topple. Thus Carter's national health insurance program, which relied upon the incremental approach to get to a universal and comprehensive national health insurance program, was a trap for liberal Democrats, and thus for him. Reforms needed to be put into place at the same time that the commitment to expand coverage was made.

The unions, much more than Kennedy, felt betrayed by Carter. They had heard Carter say what they wanted him to say and now they believed he was backing off. Kennedy, on the other hand, tended to view all such commitments as part of the political rhetoric until they became binding in actual legislation. By now compromising on the issue of a single system of health care, which could come about only through a uniform financing mechanism, Kennedy was able to keep the unions with him as he developed his new bill.

At the administration's press briefing Saturday, July 29, 1978, at which Carter's national health insurance principles were released, Califano and Eizenstat clearly revealed how difficult it had been to develop the administration's plan. Eizenstat said that all of the president's advisors involved in developing the principles found the task to be one of the "most complex issues we have ever faced." He added, "We also agree that for social programs of this magnitude we need a new approach in the 1970s. We cannot simply set in motion an entitlement program and allow it to roll along regardless of cost and administrative problems or changed economic conditions . . . We are committed to finding more intelligent ways of phasing in social programs so that their expenditures do not always exceed our initial projections."[110] Another Medicare-Medicaid program would not do, yet that is what they were afraid Kennedy would lead them to.

These statements were viewed by some as just another way Carter had of begging the issue, but Eizenstat was raising very serious concerns and ones that clearly had to be dealt with by Congress as well as the administration.

The president's goal, Eizenstat went on, was a "comprehensive national health plan, which, ultimately, will provide health coverage to all Americans," and provide the foundation upon which to build a national health plan, rather than merely a national health insurance program, thus emphasizing the need to address the issues of health cost inflation and system reform as well as providing for payment of services. But, he added, acknowledging that Carter had to view the issue in the broad context of all the problems facing the president, Carter was also committed to "solving our nation's economic difficulties, and particularly, to fighting inflation. He wants a national health plan that will help us—not hinder us—in this battle against inflation." The principles then being released offered this opportunity, Eizenstat argued.[111] They would protect the federal government from another Medicare-Medicaid episode.

In this sense, they reflected how little ground the administration had been able to cover in designing a full package. The lack of progress was only in part, though, a reflection of how difficult the task was. By that time, the summer of 1978, there were clear signs of incompetency in the Carter presidency; efforts to develop programs such as national health insurance reflected this phenomenon. Carter's inability as a leader to pull consensus out of the bureaucratic decision-making apparatus was becoming more striking, and the inability to make any significant forward motion with regard to national health insurance suggested that the final plan, when it at last came forward, would not be able to make any significant headway in Congress.

The major principles in Carter's July document included stipulations that a national health insurance plan assure that all Americans have comprehensive health care coverage, including protection against catastrophic medical expenses and assurance that all have freedom of choice in the selection of physicians, hospitals and health delivery systems. The national health plan was also to have a mechanism that would help control inflation in health care spending, including a device to contain hospital costs and strengthen competitive forces in the health care sector. The plan would require no additional federal spending for the first few years. It would be financed by government funds and contributions from employers and employees. The private insurance industry would have a significant role, with appropriate government regulation.

It was apparent that the administration was overwhelmed by the complexity of the task of designing a national health insurance plan, particularly one that would receive a sympathetic hearing from all quarters. The Carter White House was determined not to create a program that once in place would be unmanageable in a budgetary way, thus avoiding the experience of Medicare and Medicaid—issues, which at least for the moment, Kennedy did not have to worry about. The administration's strong desire not to fuel the fires of inflation obviously was a key factor in its decision to proceed cautiously and retain the possibility of approaching the task piecemeal or even aborting the plan altogether should economic circumstances dictate.

Eizenstat in a 1983 interview would say that delay until July 1978 by the Carter administration in going forward with the bare outline of its national health insurance plan was a fatal mistake. By then the economic and political climate had changed so that the proposal faced overwhelming obstacles. Not only had government been forced into a new phase—away from expansion of services and programs and into retrenchment in order to protect its fiscal beachhead—but people had become highly disillusioned with government at all levels and its abilities to solve problems and make life better.

Just a month earlier, Californians had voted to support Proposition 13, which put a limit on the state's taxing power, a vote interpreted throughout the country as strong evidence that people were fed up with the rising cost of government and its poor performance in making life better for them.

The mood of Congress changed along with that of the voters. If some members in the early days of the Carter administration were apprehensive about national health insurance, many more were apprehensive now. Thus, by the time Califano and Eizenstat met the press to explain Carter's approach to NHI, they felt they had to present a very convincing argument that the plan was workable—that it would do for people what they said it would do.

But Eizenstat, actually, felt, at least in retrospect as he described the problems of 1978 in an interview in early 1983, that the administration had missed its chance—the "window of opportunity had closed." The obstacles now were too overwhelming. The administration should have presented its national health insurance plan along with hospital cost containment early in 1977 and pushed rapidly for quick enactment—still that would have taken time. Budget deficits were rising and inflation was taking its toll.

And now, even though the principles were out, it would take even more time to develop the legislation. The fall's elections were approaching, and neither the White House nor most main-line Democrats—particularly those who were guardians of economic policy in the House, such as Ways and Means Chairman Al Ullman—wanted to have to campaign with the details of an NHI plan on the table. That put off release of the full plan until 1979.

When the negotiations between Kennedy and Carter broke down, the leaders of the citizens-labor coalition, the Health Security Action Council, which was backing Kennedy's effort, were furious, and the NHI purists on the council believed their resistance was vindicated. The episode convinced them, and Kennedy and his staff as well, that Carter was never really serious about developing a national health insurance plan and that he probably could not do it if he wanted to. The episode also added another argument to Kennedy's arsenal that Carter was not fit to be president. Both Larry Horowitz, Kennedy's aide, and Stuart Eizenstat were to say later in interviews that Kennedy would not have run against Carter in 1980 had they been able to work out an agreement on national health insurance.

There is, however, no simple answer to why they could not reach agreement. Carter of course felt that Kennedy would get the credit for NHI, and he did not want that. Kennedy increasingly believed that Carter could not be an effective president. And labor, historically and nominally still a strong backer of NHI, had many other national issues to deal with.

In 1974, health issues were not fully covered in labor contracts—particularly in auto contracts—and it was important then to labor to get these covered, if not in contracts then through a government-dictated program. By 1978, much of the coverage in the original Health Security Act was part of major labor contracts, and thus labor did not have as much to gain from enactment of a federal program, although, as noted, there would be an advantage in muting the health insurance issue in contract negotiations. The problem by 1978 was compounded by the fact that labor, and particularly the UAW, was relying on the House Ways and Means Committee, where Ullman, always resistant to NHI, was chairman, to write legislation protecting them from imports. Also, by 1978, the health care industry had expanded even further, and many of the people employed therein, particularly in hospitals but also in settling claims, were union members. Labor would have a difficult time pushing a program that would scale back the size of the industry.

When he broke with Carter in July 1978, Kennedy did not even have an outline of his own new plan ready to show to the public, but he was able to put it together in short order. In October he released the principles of his revised plan. In describing the basics of his new plan on October 2, Kennedy said he saw national health insurance

> as the last, best chance of bringing the health care system under control. It is more than a financing method. It is a system that will allow the nation to budget its health care expenses prospectively and then live within it; it is a system that will provide incentives for alternative less costly delivery models . . . it is a system that will enable, through progressive reimbursement policies, an emphasis on prevention of disease, of increasing individual responsibility for maintaining health, it is a system in which one can improve the quality of care.[112]

Soon after releasing the basics of his new plan, Kennedy held hearings at which Califano testified. While Kennedy and Carter NHI plans shared "much common ground," Califano said, there were also "some important differences." The secretary took particular exception to the proposal in the Kennedy plan that would have most of the benefit coverage in effect two years after enactment of the legislation. This should be phased in, he argued. Thus, the major difference between Kennedy and Carter seemed really to be when to start spending dollars on the program.

Califano also suggested that the Kennedy principles providing for consortia of insurance companies as the major mechanism for administering the program, and the financing scheme relying on premiums geared to each individual's earnings, were areas for potential disagreement.

The HEW secretary expressed hope that Kennedy and the administration could "work out any differences" so that together they could "build a coalition in Congress . . . with enough staying power to complete the task" of enacting a national health insurance program.[113] It was a coalition that would never materialize.

The year of all this activity, 1978, ended on a harsh note when Kennedy in December at the midterm Democratic convention in Memphis strongly criticized many aspects of Carter's domestic policy. None were more severely criticized than the failure to produce an acceptable national health insurance proposal. The climax of the two-day affair was a stirring stemwinder by Kennedy on the need for national health insurance that brought roars of approval. Two years later, of course, many of these same people would forsake Kennedy for Carter when it actually came time to name a Democratic candidate for the 1980 presidential election. Once again, national health insurance proved to be an appealing political gimmick, but when push came to shove it would drop way down on the list of political priorities.

Kennedy's principal objective at Memphis, it appeared, was to reaffirm the commitment by the Democratic Party and the Carter administration to national health insurance legislation, and to pursue that goal in the next Congress, the 96th—and that recommitment was made.

Indeed, Kennedy's reception at the midterm convention may have helped convince him that if he went after the nomination he would have substantial support from the troops of the Democratic Party. Before the conference, Kennedy was apprehensive about his participation, for he would be challenging a sitting president of his own party. After his reception there, he probably realized that such a challenge might be made successfully.

Despite this raucous debate and showmanship, as the year ended very little substance stood between Kennedy and Carter on the NHI issue, particularly compared to where they had started from. The only remaining major disagreement as expressed by Kennedy was whether the phasing-in of the program should be tied to the nation's economy and whether the proposal should be offered as single or multiple pieces of legislation. These differences between Kennedy and Carter, however, although they would attempt to get together again on a compromise, would never be resolved, and in the end failure by the two men to arrive at a compromise contributed significantly to the failure of national health insurance during Carter's term.

Carter's severe problems with national health insurance in 1978 coincided with his problems with hospital cost containment. Both issues would spill over to 1979.

Another Try at Cost Containment

As 1979 opened, President Carter prepared to push forward on two major pieces of health legislation—his national health insurance plan, the details of which he had yet to put forward, and his hospital cost-containment proposal, which he had wanted enacted by the previous Congress but which had been turned down. Now, with the 96th Congress opening, he presented a new version of hospital cost containment—one that many members of Congress had wanted him to back the year before.

As the year began, the administration was optimistic that Congress would enact the proposal, and so were some members of Congress. Speaker O'Neill early in the year said that if he could get the legislation to the floor, the House would pass it, and he set a target of early summer.

In his State of the Union address to Congress, the president reiterated the problem caused by rising hospital costs:

> A responsible budget is not our only weapon to control inflation. We must act now to protect all Americans from health care costs that are rising $1 million an hour, 24 hours a day—doubling every five years. We must take control of the largest contributor to that inflation—skyrocketing hospital costs. There will be no clearer test of the commitment of this Congress to that anti-inflation fight than the legislation I will submit again this year to hold down inflation in hospital care. Over the next five years my proposal will save Americans a total of $60 billion of which $25 billion will be savings

> in the federal budget itself. The American people have waited long enough. This year we must act on hospital cost containment.[114]

The price tag of inflation had gone up, and Carter was clearly throwing the gauntlet to members of Congress to take on the health care industry.

Two months later, on March 6, when, for the second time, he actually sent his legislation to Capitol Hill, Carter explained again why, in his view, regulatory legislation was needed to control hospital costs, although this approach was not appropriate for the rest of the economy. He said:

> In the past, hospitals have had little incentive to be efficient. The hospital sector is fundamentally different from any other sector in our economy. Normal buyer-seller relationships and normal market forces do not exist. The consumer of services—the patient—rarely pays the bill directly. Nor does the patient decide what services he or she will receive in the hospital. The person who makes those decisions—the physician—does not pay the bill either, and therefore has little or no incentive to see that services are provided in an efficient manner. Often, doctors do not even know the costs of the tests and x-rays they order.[115]

The consumer-patient was not responsible; the physician was, but could not easily be controlled; so the answer was to regulate hospitals.

Although the president got congressional health leaders to join him at the White House when he sent the new version forward, one of them, Herman Talmadge, avoided making an endorsement. In 1978, Talmadge had voted against the proposal, but by 1979 he was willing to concede that he and the president had the "same objective" in developing legislation that would restrain the rise in hospital costs. He suggested a "march in unison to the Senate this year with a good bill" that could be enacted; his idea of a good bill, though, had more of his Medicare-Medicaid reform act in it. Carter's hospital cost-containment legislation alone was not one he could endorse.[116]

Talmadge's moderation, in retrospect, however, appeared to be more a product of the impending perils of his political life than of his belief that his Medicare-Medicaid reform legislation would be improved by folding the president's hospital cost-containment bill into it. At that point, in March, the president was doing very well in his informal race against Edward Kennedy, who had not yet announced for the 1980 Democratic Party presidential nomination, while Talmadge, having been rebuked by his Senate colleagues after the seamy side of his personal life and scandal in his political life had been described in detail in the press, was facing a tough reelection battle.

The 1979 version of the bill was milder than the 1978 version. Among other changes, it carried a new first phase that gave the hospital industry a chance to meet the problem of rising costs through its own cost-cutting devices; only if that did not work would the mandatory federal regulation come into effect. This was the change Dan Rostenkowski had proposed in late 1977 and that the administration had rejected out of hand. Now the president's health policy-makers embraced the change. HEW Secretary Califano appeared before the Senate Finance Committee in support of the proposal in March, but then he was much less adamant that the president's position be adopted without change. Califano suggested that the Senate had made a commitment to this same approach the previous year when it adopted Gaylord Nelson's amendment before passing the Talmadge bill, and he acknowledged that the administration had learned a great deal.

At the same time, however, doubts were beginning to develop on Capitol Hill that the savings in Medicare and Medicaid expenses the president said would result from the bill—one of the principal arguments for its enactment—would materialize. The Congressional Budget Office in May predicted that savings from the proposal would reach only $600 million, rather than the $1.7 billion that the administration said the program would save in the next year.[117]

The Senate Finance Committee, however, never did take up the president's bill separately in 1979. Instead, it considered the measure in conjunction with its work on Talmadge's Medicare-Medicaid bill, just as it had done the year before. During its early consideration of the Talmadge bill, the panel made several tentative decisions to include parts of the president's bill, but when the telling vote was taken on July 12, 1979, the panel rejected the concept.

Russell Long, then the committee's chairman and an extremely skillful legislator, had, between the 1978 defeat of the proposal and the committee's deliberations in 1979, come to an understanding with the administration, however vaguely articulated, over national health insurance and hospital cost containment. Long wanted his catastrophic health insurance plan enacted—that was to be his contribution in this era to improving the health of the people. Catastrophic health insurance was part of Carter's NHI plan—an increasingly visible part now that the administration had gotten the message that by making it important Long would support Carter on hospital cost containment.

July 12 was a day of confusion, as had become customary for the Finance Committee. The troops of both sides were out in force. The hearing room was packed with onlookers, lobbyists, reporters and others watching the show.

Gaylord Nelson, the Wisconsin Democrat who had been the chief spokesman in the Senate for the administration's hospital cost-containment effort, after several delays was finally to put the president's plan before the committee for a vote, just as he had done the year before. Nelson, who often failed to temper his liberal bias with ingredients to attract the opposition, expounded only on the high dangers from rising health care costs and did little to describe what he believed to be the virtues of the plan he was putting before the committee.

Long, appearing restless, was clearly eager to get the vote over with; he seemed to know Nelson would lose, although he, Long, would vote with him, and he had little interest in tying the panel up further on an unwinnable issue. Finally, Robert Dole, of Kansas, then the senior Republican on the committee who two years later would become its chairman and who had been adamant in his opposition to hospital cost containment, offered a motion to table Nelson's amendment. The vote was 11–9, with Long voting in the minority and thus for the president's plan. Three years later, when chairman of the committee, Dole admitted, as the members once again struggled with ways to mitigate the rise of hospital costs on the Medicare and Medicaid programs, that he might have made his current job easier if during the Carter years he had gone along with the president's proposal. Since Talmadge was absent, Long cast his proxy, somewhat ironically, in support of Dole, giving Dole the margin he needed to win. Although Long had switched his own position from the previous year, he did not try to persuade enough other members to switch with him, and thus allowed the proposal to fail in his committee. In the end, Long would not even twist the arm of Talmadge, his long-time southern colleague, who then needed every friend in the Senate he could find. If he had done so successfully, the vote on the Dole motion would have been a 10–10 tie, and thus would have failed. The problem then would have been to get a winning vote for the Nelson amendment.

The administration and the Finance Committee continued to work toward a compromise, and finally during the summer, behind the scenes, they were able to come to terms. If the House passed a hospital cost-containment bill, the committee would be willing to accept a version that would extend to all hospital payments the essential principles of the original Talmadge bill—making a distinction between hospitals based on how efficiently they operated—rather than limiting it just to Medicare and Medicaid reimbursements. This would give the administration, in essence, what it wanted, a device to cap inflation in all hospital charges.

Meanwhile, in the House, members were also frustrated by the complexity and time-consuming nature of the measure. Ways and Means, the first panel to act, adopted a version acceptable to the administration. The Commerce Committee finally got down to work in mid-September, after a faltering effort by Henry Waxman to win approval of the measure in his health subcommittee.

Waxman, first elected to the House in 1974 as part of the post-Watergate Congress, represented part of Los Angeles. A strong liberal who had served in the California legislature before running for Congress, Waxman had been a member of the health subcommittee from the start of his congressional career. When Paul Rogers announced his retirement in June 1978, Waxman was fifth in seniority on the subcommittee and fifteenth on the full committee. When the 1978 elections were over, because of additional retirements and decisions by members senior to him to head other subcommittees, Waxman was only one slot away in seniority from the chairmanship. He sought the post and won it by getting his colleagues to choose him over Richardson Pryor, a former judge from North Carolina. But the election, which Waxman won by a 15–12 vote, left some scars. Not only did organized labor and some other members of Congress, including Edward Kennedy, lobby for him, but he relied on the goodwill he had developed in the fall when he had contributed to the campaigns of others.

Waxman's position in Congress was safe. In 1974 he won by 64 percent of the vote, in 1976 by 68 percent and in 1978 by 67 percent. Thus, by his third election, when he did not need substantial funds to win, he took contributions he received and contributed them to his own political action committee—then he made contributions to people running who shared his liberal ideology. Some of these recipients were able to vote for him as chairman of the health subcommittee in the 96th Congress. It was a tactic that had not been used before in Congress, at least by a junior member campaigning for a subcommittee chairmanship. Although Waxman won the job, he lost his liberal majority on the subcommittee. Several members who had sat on the panel the previous year moved off to take seats on other subcommittees and Waxman was left with a membership that had a strong conservative bent, including David Stockman, then a young GOP congressman from Michigan, and Phil Gramm, a very conservative Democrat from Texas who in 1983 was to switch to the Republican Party.

This group caused him difficulty all year and flatly refused to endorse any hospital cost-containment measure. Waxman thus had to take a negative recommendation to the full committee. There the votes, as in the previous year, were usually close—within one or two—so that every vote tended to be crucial. Lobbying by both the administration and the hospital industry was heavy during the five days of debate on the proposal. What promises, if any, were made by either the hospital industry or the administration remained obscure, but it was clear that both were directing the votes for at least some of the committee's members. On one amendment, Michael Bromberg, the executive director of the Federation of American Hospitals, an organization representing investor-owned hospitals, the chief strategist from the hospital industry in opposition to the proposal, standing in the rear of the room was seen to signal Jim Santini, a Democratic representative from Nevada, who had been a consistent opponent of the legislation, to switch his vote, which he did. The switch, however, did not change the final outcome of that amendment.

The most strident, and important, portions of the debate over hospital cost containment took place around the issue of allowances for increased costs due to better care, or what was called the intensity factor. The administration proposed that hospitals as part of the overall inflation target each year be allowed to increase costs 1 percent to improve capacity to deliver higher-quality health care. These additional costs often come about because of the installation of more expensive equipment.

The Carter administration sought through its cost-containment proposal to put limits on the technological advances in health care. A major portion of the increase in hospital costs, it realized, resulted from the purchase of expensive new technology such as the CAT scanner. What the Carter team was not able to do was evaluate the extent to which such advances brought improved care, and the formula in its cost-containment bill allowed for only a small increase in hospital costs annually for such improved care, or the intensity factor.

The issue had both an emotional and a fiscal grounding. It was emotional because smaller hospitals, usually those serving remote areas, did not have the most advanced technology. If hospitals were limited to a 1 percent annual increase in costs to compensate for the higher cost of improved services, it would be difficult, representatives of these hospitals argued, to install the latest equipment without exceeding the overall inflation rate for the year. Members from districts with small hospitals maintained that the provision would keep their constituents from achieving parity in health care, and thus they objected strenuously.

It was a fiscal issue because the hospital industry was undergoing tremendous technological advances, and barriers to putting those new technologies to work in hospitals hurt both the hospitals and the industry that developed the new technologies. From the administration's point of view, however, the introduction of new medical technology was a major factor in driving up health care costs.

The issue was crucial to the larger debate over the extent to which American medicine should push for the best and latest in life-saving techniques for all hospitals or focus instead on other types of health care that would have other kinds of payoffs.

The course of the hospital cost-containment bill was tortuous nearly all the way. Once approved by both the Ways and Means and Commerce committees, the measure had to go through one more panel before it could be scheduled for action on the House floor. In the House, the Rules Committee sets the debate parameters for most legislation—how long a debate and what kind of amendments, if any. Richard Bolling, then chairman of the committee, saw trouble ahead for the measure on the floor and tried to delay its arrival there to give the administration more time to strengthen its forces. The White House was pushing to get the measure onto the floor, although Bolling said he expected it would be rejected if the administration went forward with it then. The White

House had told the House leadership that if it waited until after Thanksgiving, members would be lobbied by hospital forces during the recess, and thus chances would be even poorer after that brief holiday.

Speaker O'Neill shared Bolling's estimate, but he also seemed resigned to having to defend a measure on the House floor that he knew had little chance of adoption. All year long, O'Neill had argued about the rising costs of hospital care and how unfair they were to the workingman. Indeed, until midsummer he had expressed a high degree of optimism about the chances of success for the measure, if he could only get it to the floor.

O'Neill, a portly man who had represented Cambridge and Sommerville, Massachusetts, in the House since 1953 when John Kennedy abandoned the district after election to the Senate, took the classical road to leadership, moving up through the ranks year by year as others retired, were defeated or died. He became Democratic majority leader in 1973 after the incumbent, Hale Boggs, was killed in a plane crash in the Alaskan wilderness. In 1977, when Carl Albert, who was as small in physical stature as O'Neill was large, retired, O'Neill was elected speaker.

The speaker holds a press conference almost every day the House is in session, starting fifteen minutes before the convening hour. Just before the press enters the speaker's ornate office adjacent to the House floor, the other members of the leadership confer with him, and most stay around for the press conference. O'Neill often had the habit during these press conferences of waxing philosophical, taking a reporter's question as an opportunity to expound on the virtues of the American way, particularly as made possible by the Democratic Party. During one such press conference, when he was being questioned on the hospital cost-containment bill, O'Neill described some complaints from constituents over rising hospital costs and the enormity of their bills, and then went on to describe the complaints of a banker who was objecting to ever-increasing federal taxes that were depriving him of his hard-earned money. He got the speech from this banker, he said, during a trip to Texas when he was visiting the man in his huge mansion that clearly indicated that he had substantial personal wealth. What this banker would not understand, O'Neill told the press that day, was that it was the American system that had made it possible for him to earn so much money, to be able to enjoy such a high standard of living. It was, he went on, the American system, largely developed by the Democratic Party, that made it possible for virtually everyone, regardless of origin, to go out into the world of America and earn a fortune. But it was also, he pointed out, the responsibility of the federal government to help those who were not so fortunate or lucky, and that this was what the Democratic Party was all about.

That day, November 15, 1979, as the House was about to take up the president's hospital cost-containment proposal, O'Neill was not particularly ebullient or philosophical. He saw ahead the defeat of a measure he thought important to help the little man, and he was not relishing his role in that effort.

The House took nearly the whole afternoon to deal with hospital cost containment, and the debate at times went far afield. But mostly it focused on an amendment offered by Richard Gephardt, a Democrat from Missouri. Gephardt's amendment would take out all the regulatory guts of the bill and put in its place a voluntary cost-containment program and establish a federal panel that would evaluate the effort and make recommendations about how to deal with problems in the health care industry. Similar proposals had been defeated by small margins when they were offered in both the Ways and Means and Commerce committees.

Foes of the president's bill believed it was important for them to offer a substitute that appeared to attempt to deal with the problems of hospital inflation rather than ask members simply to reject the measure. That was why Gephardt offered his amendment. Supporters of the president, however, maintained that adoption of the Gephardt proposal would make the legislation meaningless, and they were right.

A central issue in the six-hour debate was the extent to which the industry's present voluntary effort had been successful, and there the case of Gephardt and his allies was strengthened by recent hospital inflation data that showed that inflation for hospitals was running about 13 percent on an annual basis, only slightly higher than inflation in the economy as a whole, suggesting that hospitals had been able to bring their inflation in line with the rest of the economy.

Most bills coming to the House floor have only one floor manager, usually the chairman of the subcommittee in which they originated. In this instance, however, because two committees—Ways and Means and Commerce—had approved the legislation, there were two floor managers, Charles Rangel, the chairman of the Ways and Means health subcommittee, and Henry Waxman, chairman of the Commerce Committee's health panel. Rangel was the more eloquent, and angry, of the two. He saw high hospital costs as a serious threat to his Harlem constituents as well as to the nation generally, and he did not stint on his rhetoric.

Waxman, as firmly in the liberal camp as Rangel, was less emphatic during the debate, but then he had had a harder time getting the measure through committee than Rangel. While Rangel had been able to push the measure through both his subcommittee and, later, through the full committee, Waxman, because of the composition of his subcommittee, had had to give up on the measure there and pass the buck to the full committee. There he was successful, but just barely, in contrast to a year earlier when the full committee had rejected the measure, but it was clear to both Waxman and Rangel when they went onto the House floor that afternoon that the chances for enactment of the proposal were slim.

In the end, the Gephardt amendment was adopted by a sizeable 234–

166 roll-call vote. Carter's hospital cost-containment proposal was dead, although the administration made faint efforts to keep it alive.

There were many explanations for the defeat of Carter's hospital cost-containment proposal. Certainly the hospital industry lobbied very aggressively against the measure. But on balance, the proposal fell primarily of its own weight. It was, virtually everyone admitted, a very imperfect device. It created an awkward scheme that would have ultimately required separate revenue caps for each hospital subject to the mandatory program. It would have been a much stronger regulatory device for the health care sector than had been experienced before. And, as David Stockman put it when it was being debated by the full House, there no longer was the "huge inflation gap between the hospital sector and the rest of the economy. That has vanished and with it the case for this kind of hastily devised, jerry built control measure."[118]

The Carter administration's efforts to win enactment of cost-containment legislation had significant impact on its ability to bring about other changes in the health care system. But by any standard, the effort was a failure.

Lobbying on the hospital cost-containment bill was heavy all during the three years of its consideration by Congress, but the lobbying was not the reason the proposal failed—it was very poor, yet highly complicated legislation that few could understand, and there seemed to most members no compelling reason for it since, by the fall of 1979, hospital inflation was nearly in line with inflation generally. The contemporary ethic was that the votes of the legislators were for sale and they were most easily bought with money, specifically campaign contributions. After the final House vote on the bill, Common Cause, a public-interest lobbying organization, in December 1979 published a study that declared "AMA campaign contributions helped kill hospital cost containment bill." Those House members who voted against the proposal, Common Cause found, "received almost four times as much in campaign contributions from the political committees of the American Medical Association as did supporters of the cost control bill." The study detailed AMA contributions for the 1976 and 1978 elections, finding that they had a dominant influence on how members voted. It concluded: "The American Medical Association has played the central role in the determination of our nation's health policies, and political contributions are the primary source of its power."[119]

Jimmy Carter and Joe Califano in their memoirs blamed heavy lobbying against the bill as the principal reason for its defeat.

Carter argued that the primary reason he was not successful was that, "in the final showdown, Congress was flooded with money, in the form of campaign contributions from the health industry." The American Medical Association "prevailed and the American people lost. The fight for equitable health care was one of my major efforts and one of my great disappointments."[120]

Califano blamed the administration's inability to win enactment of its bill on an "effective and well bankrolled lobbying by profit making hospitals, the American Hospital Association, the American Medical Association and other segments of the health care industry. . . . "[121]

Neither fully appreciated the shortcomings of the legislation, although Carter did have the modesty to say, "There is no doubt that I could have done some things better"—an apology he reiterated throughout his book.[122]

No one apparently reported the other side of the AMA contributions picture. The Common Cause study showed that sixteen members of the House voted with Carter, although they had received $5,000 or more in AMA contributions in 1978. Among this group was Dan Rostenkowski, the Chicago Democrat who in 1978 was the chairman of the Ways and Means health subcommittee and responsible for the legislation. Both the AMA and the American Hospital Association were headquartered in Chicago.

What is more, forty-one House members voted against Carter's position even though they received very modest contributions or no contributions at all from the AMA.

Lobbying works both ways, and the administration was not without its financial resources with which to provide rewards. In fact, it was this approach by the administration that finally turned Tim Lee Carter, the senior Republican on the House Commerce health subcommittee, away from the bill. He saw the administration finally convince New Jersey Democrat Florio to support the bill by yielding on his request to have a new veterans hospital constructed in his district, and the support of organized labor was won only when the administration agreed not to have the anti-inflation provisions apply to salary increases for blue-collar hospital workers—a compromise that started the hospital cost-containment bill on a downhill roller coaster during which so many exemptions were built into the bill that even if it had been enacted it would have been largely meaningless.

The Neglected Child—Prevention

While Carter was attempting to cap hospital inflation with his cost-containment bill and to redesign the financing of health care with his national health insurance plan, he was also seeking to make the population healthier by strengthening preventive health programs.

As governor of Georgia, Carter said during his first run for the presidency, he had launched a campaign to do away with diseases that were killers and cripplers, a campaign that he maintained was dramatically successful. He would, he pledged, do the same as president. And he did focus much attention on preventive health programs once he entered the White House, but nothing was done to change the basic focus of the major federal health programs, Medicare and Medicaid, away from inpatient, acute care, toward outpatient, preventive care. Thus, prevention remained the neglected child of the health care system.

Early federal intervention into the health area was to improve preventive health services, and today the most important aspect of federal health-efforts thrust is prevention because in the long run the policy will yield the greatest benefit for the most people. In the early days of the Republic, the objective was to keep seamen with contagious diseases from exposing communities on land to those hazards. Today, one focus of prevention is wiping out, through vast immunization programs, as many of the contagious diseases as possible. Other foci include educating people to live healthy lives by not smoking, using alcohol with moderation, and getting adequate exercise. Still others include the safe use of hazardous tools and the wearing of seat belts to minimize damage from automobile accidents. Prevention is the responsibility of government because no other institution in society has the capacity to reach so much of the population.

Although the federal government's role in prevention goes back to the early days of the Republic, the current policy was created in 1962 when the Vaccination Assistance Act was signed into law. Among other things, that law authorized financial aid to states and local health agencies to carry out immunization programs aimed at protecting, primarily, children against communicable diseases.

Even though in recent years many more federal funds have been spent for health care services than for prevention, the significant improvement in the health of the nation's people has largely been the result of preventive health efforts.

The health of the American people is good. In fact, according to a 1979 HEW report, it has "never been better."[123] The great killers, such as typhoid, smallpox and other communicable diseases, by then had largely disappeared, primarily because of better sanitation, housing, nutrition and changes in life-styles, as well as immunization programs.

Preventive health programs were more important than ever because it had become possible to identify the major causes of illness and premature death. Smoking, for example, had become the single most preventable cause of death; alcohol was a factor in more than 10 percent of all deaths; occupational hazards caused up to 20 percent of all cancer mortality; and injuries caused approximately 50 percent of fatalities among young adults.

Early in his presidency, as he had said he would, Carter told HEW to mount a campaign to immunize children under 15 years of age against the six major childhood diseases—measles, rubella, polio, diphtheria, tetanus and whooping cough. The goal was a 90 percent immunization level.

By 1977, when Carter came into office, the level of immunization against these diseases, largely as a result of lack of attention on the part of the Ford administration, had fallen to such a low level that the public health was threatened by minor epidemics. By September 1979, Julius Richmond, Carter's assistant secretary for health at HEW, was able to report that the campaign had had dramatic results: It had reached the 90 percent immunization level for school-age children, except in the case of rubella.[124]

Cases of measles had declined 78 percent since 1977 and mumps by 30 percent. By the fall of 1979, no cases of diphtheria or tetanus had been reported for that year among children under 15. The number of rubella cases had dropped more than 43 percent.

During his tenure, which began in the spring of 1977, Richmond as assistant secretary increasingly concentrated his energies on prevention, on promoting better health and on developing the infrastructure to make those efforts work. Other health issues, particularly the pursuit of legislation, he left to other agencies in the department, such as the Health Care Financing Administration and the Office of the Assistant Secretary of Planning and Evaluation, or to the heads of his own subordinate agencies.

The 1979 report on health promotion and disease prevention, which was the first of its kind and the last official act of Joseph Califano as HEW secretary, put primarily on the individual the responsibility for making further progress in improving the health of the American people.

Principal among those individual responsibilities, referred to repeatedly throughout the report, were such hazards as smoking, alcohol and drug abuse, and driving without seat belts.

Smoking was the health hazard the authors considered most serious. They called "cigarette smoking . . . the single most preventable cause of death. It is clear that cigarette smoking causes most cases of lung cancer—and that fact is underscored by a consistent decline in death rates from lung cancer for former male cigarette smokers who have abstained for 10 years or more. Cigarette smoking is now also identified as a major factor increasing risk for heart attacks."[125]

That to stop smoking is the most important single step an individual can take to boost his own good health was clear. Joe Califano, a former smoker, made no bones about this, and it was part of the reason he was fired in 1979, for several southern states relied heavily on the federal subsidy for growing tobacco and they were upset by Califano's stance. But the Public Health Service every year since 1964 had published a report on the hazards of smoking, so the position was not a new one for the department's head. Smoking, the 1982 report said, was still taking an extraordinary high toll. Ronald Reagan's deputy assistant secretary for health, Everett Koop, in making public that report, said "Cigarette smoking is clearly identified as the chief preventable cause of death in our society." The report showed that approximately 30 percent of all cancer deaths were attributable to cigarette smoking. Furthermore, smoking was the major cause of lung cancer and of cancers of the larynx, oral cavity and esophagus, and smoking was a contributory factor in the development of cancers of the bladder, pancreas and kidney. Smoking, Koop said, was responsible for some 340,000 deaths annually and accounted for $14 billion in health care costs each year and over $25 billion in lost production and wages.[126]

Califano, as an activist who viewed government as the principal device for bringing about societal change, saw preventive health efforts as a revolutionary opportunity. The 1979 report was his swan song and an effort in which he said he had invested much time and concern during his tenure in office. In presenting it, he said he hoped it would "encourage a second public health revolution" and that it represented an "emerging consensus among scientists and the health community that the nation's health strategy must be dramatically recast to emphasize the prevention of disease."[127]

Califano noted that the first public health revolution against infectious diseases had resulted in a dramatic shift in the pattern of killing and disabling disease. But, he said in his introduction to the 1979 report, since 1900, when the first revolution began, "the proportion of mortality from major chronic diseases such as heart disease, cancer and stroke [had] increased more than 250 percent." Clearly, he went on:

> It makes sense in that revolution to emphasize strategies for preventing these afflictions rather than relying entirely on treating them after they have already struck. Not to find and employ those strategies would be irresponsible—as irresponsible as it would have been for our predecessors merely to alleviate the ravages of small pox and polio and cholera without attempting to eradicate them.[128]

If prevention is the more humane policy, it also makes economic sense, for the savings are substantial. By 1978, it cost the federal government about $30 million per year to operate the immunization program, but the savings reaped were several times the expenditure. Every dollar spent for prevention of polio, for example, saved $90 in treatment costs.

But if the nation's health in 1979 had never been better, there were failings as well. Infant mortality for blacks was twice as high as for whites, and health generally was not as good for blacks as for whites. The death rate for all teenagers by 1979 was increasing, and the birth rate for teenagers was still high.

In order to improve preventive health services, the Carter administration sought to improve services to population groups lacking adequate care—primarily in rural and inner-city areas.

Carter's health policy, as reflected in his health budgets, thus continued to favor the national health service corps and scholarship programs designed to get health care professionals to practice in areas lacking adequate health care. People living in these areas needed improved preventive health services. By the late 1980s, the federal government would have more than eight thousand health care professionals practicing in underserved areas, if these plans of Carter were carried out.

Other federal programs that the Carter administration, spurred on by Richmond, favored as part of its prevention policy included programs for community health centers, maternal and child health, water fluoridation, occupational health and safety, health promotion and education, the centers for Disease Control's prevention and research programs, and biomedical research.

There was another area of prevention, however, on which the Carter administration focused intensely—providing all types of health care, not just immunization, to children of poor families. Unfortunately, although probably Carter's best health program, it was never enacted, and the blame lay largely with Carter himself. The president can give his personal attention only to a very few domestic programs, and for Carter child health care was not one of them.

One of the great shortcomings of the Medicaid program was that it provided so little care to children and to pregnant women who are poor, the two groups that would yield the highest return on the investment of a fully comprehensive health care program.

Like Medicare and most private health insurance programs, Medicaid was heavily oriented toward institutional care, and because of the nature of childhood ailments a small proportion of Medicaid money was spent on children despite the fact that they constituted a significant proportion of the eligible beneficiaries. Medicaid services for pregnant women were also slim. Moreover, many poor expectant mothers, because they often did not qualify for welfare, were not eligible for Medicaid services.

The Early Periodic Screening Detection and Treatment Program, called EPSDT for short, was enacted in 1967 as part of the Medicaid program to provide more care to children, but it never worked effectively. States were concerned about the potential costs of the program, as they also were about the Medicaid program generally, if implemented fully, and resisted EPSDT on the grounds that the turnover in the welfare rolls was so rapid that many children would drop from eligibility before corrective services could be completed.

Even though EPSDT was a serious disappointment it was nevertheless an important program because it substantially changed the concept of federal support for health care for a specific group, in this case the poor. It did more than simply finance health care services. It gave responsibility to the states for actively finding poor children in need of care, assessing their needs and ensuring that the necessary services were provided. It was more a program designed to keep the beneficiaries well rather than finance treatment once they became ill. But the program was slow getting started, and in 1977, a decade after its enactment, only about 2 million children, approximately 20 percent of those eligible, were covered.

In response to the inadequacy of EPSDT, the Carter administration in 1977 proposed the Child Health Assurance Program (CHAP) that would have amended Medicaid and the EPSDT program to make additional children and pregnant women eligible for Medicaid coverage and encourage states to do more for the health of children. In 1979, CHAP did pass the House just before the session ended. In the Senate, although a more modest bill was reported in both 1978 and 1979 by the Finance Committee, the proposal, having gotten mixed up with the politics of hospital cost containment, Medicare and Medicaid reform and federal aid for abortions, was never brought to the floor.

CHAP was, in essence, a comprehensive national health insurance program for poor children and poor pregnant women and if enacted could have served as both the foundation and prototype for a broader national health program at a later date. It probably also would have done more than any other single effort to curtail, in the long run, health care costs of adults by ensuring, at least partially, that infants and children who risked poor health because of their economic status got competent health care.

NHI—The Second Round

Kennedy's Memphis attack in December 1978, when he had treated Carter so harshly, solidified the White House view that he was going after the 1980 Democratic nomination. Because of this attack, because Carter's people felt that any NHI plan enacted would work more to Kennedy's political advantage than to Carter's, and because of increasing sluggishness in the economy that would make it difficult to finance a new health plan, there was little enthusiasm in the White House for going public in 1979 with a national health insurance proposal. Some officials in the administration, particularly the economists and those responsible for the budget, felt that the president would be criticized if he offered a substantial new domestic program at the same time as he was proposing a budget that called for cutbacks in many other domestic programs, including those for health.

Finally, though, by late spring, the resistance in the White House to releasing the national health insurance plan was overcome; Carter had said he would present an NHI plan and on June 12 it was released. But Carter was the last out of the gate; he had already been upstaged not only by Kennedy, who had released the details of his plan May 14, but by Russell Long, who early in the year had begun an aggressive push to have his catastrophic health care plan take center stage.

Insurance to cover the catastrophic costs of illness is an approach that some, like Kennedy, who backed a comprehensive plan providing full care at the onset of illness or accident, argued was the worst kind of health policy. It required people to run up large bills before coverage started. But catastrophic insurance had great political and fiscal appeal. It would minimize the federal government's financial burden and provide assurance to the most politically active segment of society—the middle class who were otherwise covered for health care but were afraid of losing their financial solvency should a family member become very sick with long-term illness. Grasping this reality, Long had embraced the concept of catastrophic health insurance and for years sponsored legislation to set up such a program. In order to get additional support for the measure, Long also had his bill federalize Medicaid and in other ways increase health care for the poor. It had been this feature that won the support of Abraham Ribicoff, a Democrat from Connecticut, who was a cosponsor, and other northern Democrats.

Whatever Kennedy did or said about NHI over the years, always in the background were Long and his catastrophic health plan, and whenever the Finance Committee took up national health insurance, it always focused on the Long bill and gave only passing notice to the Kennedy proposal.

Long has been written about often as the political heavyweight in the Senate, and that he is—primarily because from 1966 through 1980 he chaired the Finance Committee, which has the broadest sweep of any Senate committee over domestic issues, and he would be expected to do so again with Democratic control of the Senate. All tax matters, including all programs that are part of the Social Security Act, are under the jurisdiction of the Finance panel. Although the Finance Committee had a health subcommittee, most of the drafting work on health legislation was done in the full committee, where Long dominated the activity.

Long was an unpredictable, mercurial person well known for designing deals that stick in the final stages of writing legislation. Almost every two years when Finance chairman he presented Congress with his grand slam, a tax bill that he brought to the floor on the eve of adjournment. It invariably had something for everybody, and often embedded deep in its bosom were a few provisions he cared about very much. They were as safe from cutting as a giant sequoia in the middle of a national park.

Although the catastrophic proposal had been on the congressional agenda for awhile, Long gave it added emphasis in 1979, perhaps because NHI was fast becoming one of the most visible, and possibly most controversial, issues in the 1980 presidential campaign.

When he introduced the legislation on February 6, Long put the issue squarely in a political context. He said the debate between Carter and Kennedy over national health insurance "set into motion the political dynamics that will finally force senators and congressmen to take sides in a highly important subject which has too long remained in the backroom bargaining state."

He noted the popular presumption that the Carter and Kennedy NHI plans would "meet head on during this Congress" with one of them winning out. But because of his legislation, Long said, the issue would not be settled as generally expected. Instead, he said, Congress would "enact something very close" to his proposal.[129]

National health insurance plans, in the last analysis, had to deal with two problems: filling the gaps in existing insurance coverage by providing insurance for those who have none or who have inadequate coverage, and attempting to control the cost of health care. And in order to win sufficient political support to be enacted, NHI plans also had to place as much of the cost of the program as possible outside the federal budget—that meant requiring employers to provide good coverage and to pay for most of it.

Long's catastrophic plan was an effort to fill the gap in health insurance created when someone was sick enough to run up big health care bills. Once in place, his plan would cover, in any one year, all health expenses of anyone once they had paid $2,000 for medical care or had been in the hospital sixty days. One version of Long's bill also made improvements in Medicaid so as to provide the poor with better health care, and it encouraged employers to improve their insurance plans for their employees, a device he adopted to win support from liberals; his primary interest, however, was the catastrophic plan. Long estimated that his program would cost about $20 billion a year. If the bill was a gap filler, it did nothing to control the cost of health care, and that was a critical weakness.

Long clearly wanted a bill, some sort of national health insurance legislation, enacted in the 96th Congress. He told Califano at a meeting on April 10, 1979, that he wanted a "bill this year" and that he was "gonna help" Carter get one, and get elected. He would, he said, compromise with the president enough to get a winnable measure.[130]

Back at the White House, negotiations were still going on with Kennedy, and on April 13 Califano and Kennedy met again. Kennedy was still adamant on a single bill; phasing would flow from that. He knew that within the Senate, and certainly in the House, there was opposition to national health insurance because of the program's cost. Ullman had repeatedly expressed his opposition to NHI to Califano and others, and thus Kennedy knew that even if he did finally get presidential support for a fully comprehensive program embodied in a single bill there was virtually no chance of having such a program come into being all at once. It would have to come in steps. There was to be one final meeting between Califano and Kennedy, on April 24, but it never materialized. Kennedy called it off, saying that labor would not compromise further.[131] Once again, Kennedy seemed to be caught in the labor vise, or was labor caught in his?

So, with no chance of reconciliation with Carter, Kennedy on May 14 revealed the details of his revised national health insurance proposal. Joining Kennedy as a cosponsor of the new plan was Henry Waxman, chairman of the House Commerce health subcommittee. As a side comment during this press conference, Kennedy said he would support Carter for the presidency in 1980; within six months he was openly challenging him for the nomination.

Kennedy's plan tackled both the NHI issues: It filled virtually all the gaps and it sought to firmly control costs. And like the other proposals, it put much of the cost of insurance on employers.

The Kennedy plan mandated insurance coverage for everyone. Employers would have to provide insurance for employees and their dependents. The federal government would provide insurance for the poor, the aged, the disabled and the unemployed through a revised and upgraded Medicare program. Those otherwise not covered would be insured under the revised Medicare plan.

Everyone would have full coverage for inpatient and outpatient hospital services, physician services both in and out of the hospital, home health services, X rays and lab tests. Pre- and post-natal care would be fully covered, as would all physical examinations for children to age 18. For all those 18 years and over, routine physicals would not be covered.

A bipartisan federal authority would certify and regulate insurance companies and organizations delivering health care, which in order to receive payments from the program would have to operate under one of five national health care consortia—Blue Cross-Blue Shield, commercial insurers, health maintenance organizations, individual practice associations (a type of prepaid plan), and those companies that insured themselves. Each consortium would collect the insurance premiums and distribute them to participating members according to a predetermined annual budget. Within limits, people would be able to select the insurance program they wanted from the appropriate consortia. Hospitals would be told how much they could take in and how much they could spend annually. Doctors' fees would also be set in advance each year.

Insurance for workers would be financed through contributions by both employers and employees. Insurance for the aged, poor and unemployed would be financed by a trust fund to which workers and business would also contribute. Workers would pay up to 35 percent of the cost of insurance, but this would be their only cost—there would be no deductibles or coinsurance.

The new Kennedy program was expensive. In its first year, it would require $40 billion more for health care expenditures than was being spent nationally at that time. The federal share of the additional cost would amount to $28.6 billion; the nonfederal share, which would mostly come out of the pockets of employers and to a lesser extent those of workers, would be $11.4 billion. Four years later, the program, according to Kennedy's estimates, would result in lower expenditures for health care than the nation would spend if his new health care plan were not enacted.[132]

Kennedy's plan tackled squarely the two central issues of any NHI proposal—filling the gaps and controlling costs. But for many it was too massive and expensive a program, and besides it was not one that Russell Long would consider seriously—it wasn't in the running.

Henry Waxman, although he had not been an advocate of national health insurance, joined Kennedy in supporting the new plan because, he said later, he believed Kennedy was seriously trying to create a package that would bring about some badly needed reforms in the health care system. Carter's sincerity toward this end, from Waxman's point of view, was in doubt. Carter, Waxman believed, did not want to compromise with Kennedy. But he also said in a 1983 interview that he was cautious about radical changes, that he wanted to study the problem further and proceed slowly, which in one sense ran contrary to his support of the 1979 NHI bill. Perhaps that contradiction was explained by his acknowledgment that his stable of natural supporters—including labor—was much the same as Kennedy's and that Kennedy had supported him in 1978 when he had campaigned for the chairmanship of the health subcommittee.

Carter finally released the details of his plan on June 12, nearly a year after he had announced its basic ingredients, but it was not without some disruption within the administration that the decision was finally made to go forward. As Califano and his staff at HEW refined the plan, they found that it would cost, according to their projections, more than the budget-makers at the Office of Management and Budget wanted—about $17 billion in additional costs as opposed to the $10 billion OMB had expected. In fact, Carter wanted to cancel the announcement because of the extra cost, but Califano persuaded him that it was too late—the press conference had been publicly scheduled. Besides, Califano said, they could probably reduce the cost somewhat by making minor adjustments in the proposal. But the costs remained unchanged, and the program did go forward. All this was happening as Carter was about to retreat to his mountain top at Camp David for several weeks, after which he would descend and speak to the country about the malaise of the American people, and then fire Califano.

Carter clearly hoped that the June 12 announcement would provide the momentum needed to get some forward motion on the proposal. Surrounding him on the stage of the auditorium in Room 450 of the Old Executive Office Building next to the White House as he made his presentation were key congressional leaders: Senators Russell Long, Abraham Ribicoff and Gaylord Nelson and Representatives Harley Staggers, James Corman and Charles Rangel. Conspicuously absent were Herman Talmadge, Carter's fellow Georgian, from the Senate, and Al Ullman and Henry Waxman from the House.

The combination of attendees and absentees was revealing. Long, the chairman of the Finance Committee through which the legislation would have to pass, and Ribicoff, the ranking Democrat but one on that panel, were, as noted, sponsors again in 1979 as they had been since the early 1970s of their own form of NHI focusing on catastrophic insurance. Support by Ribicoff, a liberal who had served as John Kennedy's first secretary of Health, Education and Welfare, and who for years had acted as a leader in the Senate on social, welfare and health issues, gave Carter a dimension of political oomph that was important to counteract Kennedy's opposition. But Ribicoff, as strong a liberal as he had been in the past, was losing steam. At 69, he was getting ready to retire in 1980, and although he would strongly support Carter's national health plan, he would not be able to be the catalyst to put together a winning combination. When it came his turn to speak, Ribicoff struck a theme he would repeat later during committee deliberations on the measure. "I think this is doable this year," he said, but the effort needs the cooperation of all "the main actors," President Carter, Senators Kennedy and Long; "there is no reason why" they "can't compromise these differences or work them out."[133]

Ribicoff's leader on the panel, Russell Long, had different reasons for giving Carter support at this opening effort. A populist from Louisiana, whose consistency and integrity were constantly in question because of the erratic way he pursued his legislative responsibilities, Long was probably ideologically incapable of finding compatibility with Ted Kennedy. Whatever chance there was for such an accommodation may have evaporated in 1969 when Kennedy had ousted Long from the job of Senate Democratic whip by a 31–26 vote. It left a bitter scar with Long, the salve for which sometimes was to retaliate against Kennedy in ways that could hurt the Massachusetts senator. One of those ways was to undermine Kennedy's national health insurance effort. Two years later, in 1971, Long had gotten some vicarious satisfaction when another conservative, Robert Byrd, defeated Kennedy for the whip job by a 31–24 vote. That ouster was probably due in part to Kennedy's demonstrable lack of interest in the nuts and bolts of the whip job, but as much or more it also perhaps reflected disenchantment by Senate Democrats with Kennedy for his role in the Chappaquiddick incident in the summer of 1969. That incident, in which Kennedy caused the death through drowning of a young woman as the result of an automobile accident, would plague Kennedy for the rest of his political career. Some argued that at least through 1980 it had been a cause, as much as any other reason, for the failure of national health insurance to win enactment, because it had been a major reason Kennedy had not run for the presidency.

When it came his turn to speak during Carter's presentation of his NHI plan, Long said he applauded the president for "providing leadership. . . . We on the Finance Committee will study the president's recommendations. We'll add some of our own . . . and bring the Senate a bill," he said, and emphasized that as far as he was concerned it was entirely possible to negotiate a successful compromise.[134]

Gaylord Nelson, like Ribicoff, might have bridged the gap in the Senate between liberals and conservatives, not because he had much rapport with conservatives (as somewhat of a maverick liberal he often caused chafing by conservatives), but because he sat on both the Labor and Human Resources health subcommittee, which Kennedy chaired, and Long's Finance Committee. In addition, Nelson was the administration's chief spokesman for hospital cost containment in the Senate. Nelson, too, would be leaving the Senate at the end of 1980, but not on his own initiative. He would be defeated in his reelection effort, one of a number of Democratic defeats that would turn the Senate in 1981 over to the Republicans for the first time in twenty-six years.

The support of Jim Corman, a liberal Democratic representative from Los Angeles, for Carter's national health plan was important because Corman not only sat on the Ways and Means Committee but, more important, for many years had been cosponsor with Kennedy of the Health Security Act. Now, however, he had broken with Kennedy to support Carter because Kennedy's new plan violated a principle he thought very important: It would use federal funds to purchase health insurance in the private sector for the poor and aged. He believed strongly that federal funds should be more closely managed by the federal government. Corman, too, would be defeated in 1980 as the House became more conservative in advance of Ronald Reagan's presidency.

Charles Rangel, another liberal Democratic member of Ways and Means, was chairman of that panel's health subcommittee, which would have partial responsibility for national health insurance in the House. Rangel also was the only black among the group to be sponsoring Carter's plan. Harley Staggers, a former sheriff of Mineral County, West Virginia, and in 1979 chairman of the House Commerce Committee, was a mild-mannered man who more often than not seemed overly concerned about not offending others but he often faded into the background and was forgotten. Indeed, when Carter was asking each of the members present to comment on the proposal he forgot to seek out Staggers's remarks and had to be reminded by Califano, who whispered in his ear, to do so.

The absent House members, Ullman and Waxman, were important because Ullman chaired the Ways and Means Committee and Waxman the Commerce health subcommittee. Since Commerce and Ways and Means shared jurisdiction over national health insurance, their lack of support for the Carter proposal suggested that the measure would have a hard time generating momentum, and interest, in the House. Ullman, a moderately conservative member and a lackluster leader who would lose his seat in the 1980 election, was sponsoring other national health insurance legislation, a proposal geared around schemes to make the national health care system more competitive. Waxman, as noted, earlier in the year had joined as a cosponsor of Kennedy's health care act for all Americans.

Talmadge, the highest-ranking Democrat on the Finance Committee after Long, chairman of its health subcommittee and Carter's fellow Georgian, never had shown much interest in national health insurance. His main piece of health legislation—the proposal to reform Medicare and Medicaid—had been rejected by Carter soon after his inauguration in 1977 in favor of his hospital cost-containment plan. But Carter would need Talmadge if his health insurance legislation was to be successful.

Although the centerpiece of Carter's plan was a scheme to provide protection against the high costs of very expensive medical care, it was more than a catastrophic health insurance plan. It would also, he argued, make modest improvements in health care coverage for the elderly and disabled and broaden coverage for the poor. The Carter health plan would cost only an estimated additional $17 billion in federal expenditures in its first year, but, he said, in describing his new plan, passage at the same time of hospital cost containment was a must.

In presenting the plan, Carter said:

> A universal comprehensive health program is among the great unfinished items on our nation's social agenda. The national health plan I am proposing today establishes the framework and creates the momentum to reach that long sought goal. In future years, the plan can be expanded to include all low income persons. Employer coverage can be made more fully comprehensive with subsidies to ease the burden on small businesses. First dollar coverage for preventive services can be extended throughout early childhood . . . These expenditures are a social investment in the future of our children, the economic security of our elderly, and the well being and peace of mind of all Americans. They are an investment in a more effective and efficient health care system. Over time, the plan's emphasis on prevention, competition and cost containment will reap important dividends for our nation and its people.[135]

It was, conceptually, a very attractive plan, for it allowed a modest takeoff, thus responding to the concerns of those alarmed by the Medicare-Medicaid experience, yet offering to others the expectation, ultimately, that a fully comprehensive plan could come into being.

But it dealt only partially with the two basic NHI issues—it filled some gaps and it controlled costs to a certain extent. Virtually everyone would have health insurance in one way or another under Carter's plan, and the cost of very expensive illnesses would be covered, but the benefits, at least in the initial stages, would be more limited than under Kennedy's plan and health care costs would not be as tightly controlled. Its ability to control costs depended on passage of the hospital cost-containment proposal, which a few months later was to be permanently laid to rest, and only a partial limit on physician fees—those paid for through the public program. Most physician expenses would be paid for through the private health insurance system, and those would not be affected by the Carter plan.

The plan had two parts—one for those who were already beneficiaries of Medicare and Medicaid, which Carter called Healthcare, and a second for the employed. Each was primarily a catastrophic program, although the definition of when the "catastrophe" struck was different for each group covered. The poor would get all their care free. The elderly and disabled would pay some of the cost of care until they had spent $1,250—the catastrophic limit. For workers, the catastrophic cut-off was $2,500. Individuals not eligible for coverage through their jobs could purchase insurance separately, and those who could not purchase coverage from private insurance carriers at a reasonable rate would be eligible to buy into Healthcare.

The major benefits required by the Carter plan, both under Healthcare and the employer-sponsored plans, included unlimited hospital inpatient services for acute care, prenatal, delivery, postnatal and total infant care through the first year, unlimited physician and other ambulatory services (including laboratory and X rays but excluding dental coverage), 100 days each of skilled nursing care and home health visits each year, 20 days of inpatient psychiatric care per year plus $1,000 worth of outpatient services, and preventive services for persons through age 17.

Physicians participating in Healthcare would be required to accept predetermined fees for each type of service. But the limitations on physician fees applied only to Healthcare beneficiaries, not to fees charged to beneficiaries of employer insurance plans or other patients, creating the potential for a two-tiered health care system—a shortcoming its opponents were quick to point out. Hospital charges would be limited by the hospital cost-containment bill, the one that was soundly rejected by the House. Carter's Healthcare plan would be financed by payroll taxes and general revenues. The cost of the program not met through the existing Medicare payroll tax would be financed out of general revenues.

Although the administration contended that the national health plan contained devices to stimulate competition, these devices were limited. Employers would be required to provide coverage through a health maintenance organization, if one was available in the area, and Healthcare participants would be encouraged to use HMOs. Building on the precedent established in the 1977 law that permitted Medicare, under some circumstances, to pay for the care given the elderly by health care professionals who were not physicians, Healthcare would pay for services provided by clinics, nurse practitioners and specialized treatment centers in addition to services provided by physicians. In this way, the administration hoped to stimulate further competition between providers. The only other such device, however, would apparently be competition between businesses seeking the job of processing Healthcare claims.

Once in place, phase one of the administration's national health plan would relieve state and local governments of about $2 billion in health care costs annually, according to White House estimates, by decreasing their share of Medicaid costs and providing health care services to low-income individuals.

Following Carter's presentation on June 12, HEW Secretary Califano, describing the plan further, made a point of emphasizing that there were only three essential differences between the Carter and Kennedy plans. The Kennedy plan required premiums related to income, whereas under the Carter plan premiums would be determined by the program through which the individual was covered. The Kennedy plan also would force insurance companies to work through one of four consortia, while the Carter plan would rely on the insurance industry essentially as it was presently arranged. Furthermore, Kennedy's plan called for enactment of the entire program at once, while Carter would have his program enacted in several phases over a number of years.

A central difference overlooked by Califano was the requirement in the Kennedy proposal for an annual budget for the nation's health care bill, a principle that Carter in the past had strongly endorsed but which was absent from the plan as presented in the summer of 1979. Administration officials contended that prospective budgeting would come about through enactment of hospital cost-containment legislation, but that would apply only to hospitals and then only to those subject to the program.

In addition to the three Democratic plans—Carter's, Kennedy's and Long's—Republicans in the Senate had one as well. Three members of the Finance Committee—Robert Dole, John Danforth and Pete Domenici—sponsored a less generous catastrophic proposal that started coverage only after an individual had paid $5,000 in medical expenses. Employers would be required to provide catastrophic coverage to workers, Medicare would get a catastrophic lid, states would be required to add catastrophic coverage to Medicaid and a fourth plan would be created for the uninsured. Employers would not have to pay more than 25 percent of the cost.

Even if President Carter wanted only a limited national health insurance program enacted during the first round, he did have plans for a larger, more comprehensive one that would be enacted in future years, although there was no schedule for when the additional elements would be proposed or when he wanted them to be operational.

The larger program would build upon the two key elements of the initial proposal—Healthcare and the employer-based plan—and it mandated a broader range of services. It would include unlimited hospital, physician and diagnostic services, and specific but limited amounts of coverage for other types of care, including skilled nursing care, home health care, mental health services, and prescription drugs. In addition, the free prenatal, pregnancy and postnatal care for children through the first year of life mandated in the first phase would be expanded, ultimately, to extend through age six.

Besides expanded benefits of services, the ultimate Carter plan would have expanded financial benefits. Cost sharing would be modified so that all deductibles (the fee paid before coverage starts) would be eliminated and coinsurance (except for all care through age six that would continue to be free) would be set at 25 percent. Catastrophic coverage would be improved. The definition of "poor" would be broadened somewhat so that the group receiving all care without cost would be expanded.

The larger program would be financed, as would the initial phase, by the Medicare payroll tax and by requiring employers to pay at least 75 percent of the premiums of health insurance for their employees. Health care for the poor provided through the public program would be paid for out of general revenues of the Treasury.

Under the expanded, future Carter health plan, the cost of health care would be contained by the same devices to be used in the first phase of the program—primarily by the yet-to-be-enacted hospital cost-containment program and by limits on physicians fees under Healthcare. While the physician-fee schedule would not apply to charges for care to patients covered by private insurance, the White House said in describing the fully comprehensive plan that it expected the federal schedule to have an effect on fees for services outside of the public system. If it did not, the administration would propose legislation setting fee schedules for all physician care. People would be encouraged to use health maintenance organizations as a way of cuting the cost of care. The administration said that if the devices it proposed did not hold in line the rise in health care costs, it would consider establishing a national health budget. That feature had been endorsed by Carter in his April 1976 speech to the black medical students and was a central feature in Kennedy's plan, but it was a politically risky proposal and therefore should be pushed only as a last resort.

There was, as noted, a striking similarity between the Carter plan, at least the initial phase, and that proposed by Richard Nixon in 1974. But once Carter had rejected the full package contained in Kennedy's Health Security Act and a much simpler and cheaper catastrophic health insurance plan advocated by Russell Long, there was not much else he could do in the middle area that would not resemble Nixon's plan. The essential element of the Nixon-Carter approach was to run as much of the cost of the program through the private sector by mandating that employers purchase health insurance with prescribed benefit levels for their employees. To what extent the cost of that coverage was paid for by the employee or employer made no difference in terms of the costs to the federal government.

The Senate Finance Committee was the only committee to make substantive progress on the development of a national health insurance proposal in 1979. It was Long who was orchestrating the progress and obviously enjoying it.

Appearing before that panel on March 27, 1979, before the details of the Carter plan had been released, Califano rejected Long's "catastrophic only" approach and described the yet-to-be-announced Carter plan as one that could go beyond catastrophic insurance and "seek to improve coverage for all segments of the population—the aged, the poor, the employed and others—and will seek to put in place new structures that will require only future expansions for the realization of President Carter's goal of universal, comprehensive plan."[136]

Despite that position, Long, who coveted his own catastrophic bill, said that although he and the president might disagree on "an ultimate plan for complete national health insurance . . . we can certainly reach agreement on this important [first] step."

Long indicated that he wanted to move quickly with a catastrophic health insurance program. He said he intended to "push for the earliest possible implementation of this most crucial element of care." But, he added:

> I would also like to work with the president in assuring that we have in place proper controls in the areas of technology assessment, professional oversight and approval of capital expenditures. One of my own disagreements with the president's plan is not one of substance, but of timing. I understand that the president's plan would allow no new federal spending before 1983, but I see no reason to hold back on the catastrophic health insurance part of the program. Illness and injury just don't wait until convenient times.[137]

In June, Long made a statement on the Senate floor outlining his position on NHI and predicting Senate action on a bill his committee would report, soon. An NHI program, he said, should provide catastrophic health insurance protection against the costs of "very serious and very expensive illness and injury." This was where he agreed with Carter, and it was a matter of principle. But he and Carter disagreed over how extensive that coverage should be, and therefore how costly, and when it should become effective. The poor, he and Carter agreed, should be adequately covered, and standards should be set for private health insurance policies. The insurance industry should be relied upon to the fullest extent possible, and public financing should be kept to a minimum.

Long's differences with Carter (and with Kennedy) arose when developing the next phase, the program that would be enacted after the initial one that was to be enacted in 1979. The Senate, he said, would not enact Kennedy's cradle-to-the-grave bill, for there were "powerful elements" opposing it.[138]

No sooner had the president released the details of his national health plan than Long's Finance Committee went back to work on the measure, with an emphasis on compromise and accommodation.

When the panel convened on June 19, Long began a series of combined drafting and hearing sessions. Long, then, was clearly of a mind to move forward, and to get out of committee a national health insurance proposal as soon as possible. In part, this had to do with Long's restless nature and intolerance for tedious, drawn-out sessions and in part due to his realization that momentum was developing and that he needed to grasp and capitalize on that if the 96th Congress was to turn out some sort of national health insurance program.

As the panel convened at 9:15 A.M. in its regular meeting room on the second floor of the Dirksen Senate Office Building, other members of the committee, too, were talking about compromise and accommodation; it seemed within their grasp. In his opening remarks, Long stressed that "we ought to try, in my judgment, to make progress and headway in this area." Ribicoff than stepped in, fulfilling his role as both accommodator and synthesizer. "I think that we have before us today a great opportunity to finally have a health insurance plan," he said. "Frankly, I think it is going to be along the lines advocated by you (Mr. Chairman) and myself, but for the first time you have the president of the United States and Senator Kennedy with their proposals, which look to me that they have basically adopted some of the philosophies that you originally advocated."[139]

But then Ribicoff threw cold water on Long's approach when he went on to describe the task of the committee, as he saw it, in working its way through the various proposals—economic impact, systems reform, subsidies to employers, benefit package, cost controls, limits on construction of new health care facilities, controls over utilization of health care services, and more—that for the committee to start writing a bill "without knowing what we are talking about, I think would be self defeating." He continued:

> I really, truly believe that we can pass national health insurance and I think we are going to have to give Congress and the people of this country the feeling that we have been thoughtful and careful, as we have on every major piece of legislation. I think what you have before you today, Mr. Chairman, in many ways is the most significant social and economic piece of legislation presented in the last decade, for sure, before this Congress.[140]

But it was at this point, essentially, that Ribicoff and Long parted ways, for while trying to spur on the momentum and interest that Long was showing, Ribicoff nevertheless was siding with those on the committee advocating a more cautious approach. Long had said on several occasions that he wanted to write the bill and then find a way to pay for it. His colleagues, almost universally, wanted to have some idea of what the costs would be and how those costs might be met before they were willing to commit themselves, and the Senate, to such a substantial new undertaking.

Later in the session that day, after Hale Champion, the undersecretary of HEW, testified on the president's newly released plan, Long became a witness before his own committee, and described and advocated adoption of his proposal. He was followed in the witness chair by the ranking Republican on the panel, Robert Dole. It was a session during which many national health insurance plans spilled forth, some understandings were achieved, but no lasting accommodation was arrived at.

Long's frustration began to show. He wanted to start having votes, and he wanted some action. Early in the session he, in effect, called for a vote, one way or the other, although a formal vote was never taken. "As far as I am concerned," he said, "do whatever you want to do about my suggestion" that would be offered later. "As far as I am concerned," he went on, "just vote one way or the other—yes or no, or any shade of maybe." He described the "enormous tax bills" that the committee had worked on in the past and how many more problems there were in them than in the pending proposals. "My thought," he added, "is that we sometimes have had to make some decisions to see what direction we were going to head in, otherwise we would not have had any bill, and we would still be arguing about what we should do."[141]

And Long, who would have to run for reelection in 1980, let his colleagues and the audience have it with his double whammy. He said:

> We will go before the public next year. If we do not act, many poor people will die in the meantime, and many middle income people will die in a catastrophic illness situation, or their resources will be wiped out. People will say, "Well, you talked all these years. Now, we have had six years of conversation about your plan to help these people. Why don't you ever do something up there?"[142]

It was Long's attempt to put faces before the committee members, faces of individuals, of constituents, who were suffering and would die unless the committee, and Congress, acted. But it is extremely difficult to raise the specter of dying faces when they are just a hypothetical, statistical circumstance. Earlier, in 1972, when Congress was considering enactment of the end-stage renal disease program, legislators were able, as we shall see, to bring to mind the faces of people who were desperately in need of financing for their care and who would die without it. These people had been before congressional committees and told of their plight. One had, in fact, undergone dialysis while testifying in a committee hearing room. But there were no such dramatic situations for Long to bring before the Finance Committee in the summer of 1979.

Long was trying to get some sort of serious deliberation going on the development of a national health insurance program, either in or out of the committee room. He called for a caucus of members of each party, and a few days later when Kennedy appeared before the panel he was to get him to agree, at least in principle, to the need for accommodation. But in the end it would not be possible to achieve that goal, for one very essential ingredient in the mixture would quickly evaporate. The presidency of Jimmy Carter was unraveling, and without the force of the presidency behind a proposal as complicated as national health insurance, it would not be able to move through the congressional labyrinth.

It was Kennedy's turn on June 21 to give the Finance Committee the details of his new national health insurance proposal, and he did it with his usual style. Kennedy always attracts a large audience, and in this case the committee managers reserved a separate room for the overflow crowd into which they piped the proceedings. Kennedy arrived followed by his usual phalanx of aides and a string of public witnesses who would testify about their organizations' support for his new plan. The television cameras and klieg lights were there, and Kennedy produced a set of charts and used them as a device for a virtuoso performance that dazzled the audience and the committee alike, including the chairman. Long watched Kennedy as he flipped his charts, in obvious command of the proposal he was advocating. Long sat in his chairman's seat, leaning back, gazing somewhat starry eyed at the charts and at Kennedy, like a small boy watching his idol shine. It was a startling moment during a relationship that had endured so much enmity.

As on virtually all other occasions, Kennedy dwelt on the need for reforms in the health care system, particularly on how providers are paid. Essentially, he argued for a health budget that would set limits to the amount that could be spent on health care in a given year. Without such limits, he argued, health care costs would continue to rise dramatically, every new technology would be introduced into the health care field, raising the costs even higher, and soon the new system would be out of control, just as the present one was. But it was a complicated proposal and often difficult to fathom. In this way, it was markedly different from Long's proposal, which for all its deficiencies had a simplicity that made it possible for people to comprehend, and thus be willing to live with.

As the session was drawing to a close, Ribicoff again put the whole matter in perspective:

> My feeling is, personally, that this is not going to work . . . unless Senator Kennedy has a piece of the action. . . . And I think it is not going to work unless Senator Long has a piece of the action, and I do not think it is going to work unless President Carter has a piece of the action, and Senator Dole. But it is doable, and I think that it would be a tragedy when you have reached the stage where those people can make this thing work that we allow ourselves to get involved in personalities or political one-upsmanship

to prevent it from working. I think everybody that is involved here has a great obligation to try to work this out together.[143]

Long threw this one off by saying that he was prepared to have anyone else take credit for it, and then to conclude the session—but speaking more for Kennedy than anyone else—Long said, "Let me say this as chairman speaking for the committee, that we welcome all the advice that members of this group and their associates can bring us. . . . We will try to bring out a bill that we hope the Senate will pass," and he asked if Kennedy was willing to work out such a bill. Kennedy said he was; that he had a keen desire to work with the committee, with the president and others.[144]

The Finance Committee had one more drafting session before turning to hospital cost containment, but by that time the two issues were becoming thoroughly intertwined; it was apparent that one would not go to the Senate floor without the other. On June 28, as the Finance panel was again considering the measure, the matter of coverage for children came up. It was to be an expensive proposition. Long was cautious, suggesting they wait until later to consider it. "We're going to come to the end, then see what we should do for the poor and then see how much it would cost," he said.[145]

By the end of June, Long had put off further work on national health insurance legislation until the fall, and while some work was done in the autumn months, work then was again postponed until the new session of Congress, which would start in January 1980.

In the meantime, Joseph Califano was fired from his job at HEW. The event occurred on July 18, 1979, and no one was really surprised. By that time he had become an extremely controversial character. Califano was viewed by most as abrasive, arrogant, demanding and abusive. He was viewed by some as brilliant and the most creative secretary the department had ever had. Few had neutral feelings about him.

From the point of view of most in the White House, even those sympathetic to him, Califano was out of control, and regardless of what President Carter might do to rein him in, it would have little impact. Califano believed the presidency should be run as Lyndon Johnson had run it, when Califano, in the Johnson administration, served as chief spokesman on domestic issues. Califano clearly had disdain for Carter.

Califano was selected for the HEW job after Carter's first choice, Leonard Woodcock, had turned it down. Shortly thereafter, Woodcock retired from his job as president of the United Auto Workers and Carter sent him to China, where he negotiated the normalization of the relationship between the two countries. Thus, Woodcock was not only out of his union post during the critical period of formulation within the Carter administration over national health insurance, but he was also out of the country and far away from where he might be of use to advocates of the Kennedy plan.

Carter felt a commitment to Woodcock personally on the issue of national health insurance, more than he did to organized labor and the UAW generally. Woodcock had personally campaigned for Carter in Florida in advance of the May 1976 primary, and winning that primary had been crucial for Carter. Thus with Woodcock's departure from the scene, Carter felt less strongly about his commitment on national health insurance. Had Woodcock in fact taken the HEW job, the story of Carter and national health insurance might have been much different.

The Retirement of Categorical Health Programs

While the Senate Finance Committee was attempting to come to terms with Carter's national health insurance proposal, the stage was being set, elsewhere in the administration, for bringing to an end the era of federal grant programs designed to address specific health problems.

One of Carter's early high hopes in the health area had been for the community mental health centers program; he anticipated that with his wife's interest in the field he could build a new national mental health services program that would bring credit to his administration, just as it had to John Kennedy's. But mental health no longer had the pizazz that it had had during the Kennedy years.

Throughout its history the centers program found strong support in Congress, even when opposed by the Nixon White House, but it was not seen as successful by all. In 1973, a Nader study group found that the community mental health centers program was "vastly oversold" and the original goal of the availability of efficient, effective care in every community "quickly perverted." The Nader group laid the primary responsibility for the program's failure, as it saw it, on the inability of the National Institute of Mental Health to adequately use its resources and imagination to make the program work.[146] Shortly thereafter, another study pointed out that centers were unable to provide sufficient care to those who were being discharged from state mental hospitals during an era when states were reducing the patient populations in—and sometimes closing—their mental hospitals. Many people during the 1970s were discharged because the hospitals were not treating them for their mental illness, but rather serving only as a place to live, and often not a very desirable place at that. Courts and public pressure forced their discharge into communities that were also ill equipped to provide support services—help in coping with the fundamentals of living: food, shelter, and the rest—that the state hospitals had provided, however inadequately. The logical device to fill that need was the community mental health center, but in most cases it did not have the resources to do so. The report, by the American Federation of State, County and Municipal Employees, the labor union that represented blue-collar workers in state mental hospitals whose jobs were threatened when patients were moved out of institutions, helped to chip away further at the invincibility of the centers program.[147]

In 1978 another group found that community mental health centers had serious shortcomings, so serious that the program should be abolished. This was the President's Commission on Mental Health created by President Carter soon after he entered the White House in 1977. The conclusion was largely politically contrived and sprang from the need to have a recommendation that proposed an entirely new Carter mental health program.

The commission grew out of Mrs. Carter's longstanding interest in mental health problems. As first lady of Georgia, Rosalynn Carter became deeply involved in the state's mental health programs. During the campaign of 1976 she pledged that, once in the White House, she would head a presidential commission to study these problems and search out ways federal policy in this area might be improved. But the commission also grew out of Mrs. Carter's need to have a substantive role in the administration as first lady, for she was not one to sit around the tea table.

If mental health was to be a convenient vehicle for Mrs. Carter, little, if any, thought was given to the consequences that might flow from the commission's work, and really, indeed, whether such an examination was needed. The commission, regardless of the packaging it finally had, was first of all a vehicle for Mrs. Carter to ride and, second, one which would produce a health program that would carry the Carter stamp exclusively. And because Mrs. Carter would be in charge of it, the budget ramifications about which the president was particularly concerned (he did not want an expensive, new program), the final recommendations could be kept modest. Public-interest groups, led by the National Association for Mental Health, on whose board of directors Mrs. Carter had sat prior to 1977, were eager to have the commission established and gave little thought as to what the consequences might be. Like all advocates for special-interest causes, lobbyists for mental health—and perhaps particularly mental health because of its generally uphill struggle to be accepted as a mainstream health care—were eager to have the visibility that would flow from a presidential commission.

The campaign pledge was redeemed in February 1977 when President Carter signed an executive order creating a twenty-member presidential commission to help him "achieve some progress in the field of mental health."[148] The explicit charge to the commission initially was to determine who among the mentally ill were poorly served and how the federal government could most effectively support their treatment. The implicit charge was to present the president with a modest program for federal support of mental health services that could be implemented successfully during Carter's term.

The commission, once it concluded its deliberations in 1978, found many positive results had flowed from the community mental health centers program. Before it came into being, 75 percent of those receiving mental health care were residents of state mental hospitals. By 1978, however, largely due to the centers program, that figure had been reversed and 75 percent of those receiving mental health care were by then being treated in outpatient facilities. By October 1978, there were 647 centers in operation and another 71 ready to go into operation. The number of people in state mental hospitals, the Carter commission found, had been reduced by more than half, dropping from 550,000 in 1955 to 200,000 in 1975.[149]

But still, the report concluded, state hospitals continued to provide a major portion of long-term care for the chronically mentally ill. It was on this group that the Carter commission focused part of its attention. It also found that many people with specialized needs, such as children, adolescents and the elderly, were not receiving adequate care through the community mental health centers program.

Getting mental health centers to provide a total package of care had been one of the most difficult tasks for managers at the National Institute of Mental Health, and for those outside government, such as lobby groups, concerned about the program's success. Centers tended to focus on the needs of the dominant population that they served. CMHCs in suburban areas dealt with the mental health problems of the middle class; those in urban ghettos with the problems of the poor. Often the problem of the chronically mentally ill and of children, both of whom were usually difficult to treat, were given short shrift because of shortages of staff and other resources, or simply because of the laziness of program administrators. It was on this shortcoming that the president's commission focused. It decided that funds for the mentally ill should be directed at the groups with the most need. In so doing, the commission undermined the principle—its attempt to provide all the mental health services a community could need—that made the program rare among federal health programs.

The requirement that each center have a full range of services within its comprehensive package in order to begin receiving federal funds, the commission found, "excluded many communities that needed services immediately but did not and may never require the array of services mandated by legislation. A way must be found for unserved and underserved communities to have mental health services without forcing them to assume the formidable responsibility of providing the full range of services."[150]

The commission's final report, released in April 1978, proposed creating a new federal grant program for providing community mental health services designed to correct the faults, as perceived by the commission, of the existing program. Ultimately it would replace the existing program of grants to CMHCs. The commission's recommendations, somewhat reworked by Congress, became law in 1980.

In 1981, President Reagan signed another CMHC act, when he approved the omnibus budget reconciliation act. That measure turned the CMHC and related drug and alcohol treatment programs over to the states, and so an effort that had begun fifteen years earlier to force the states to change their way of delivering care to the mentally ill was in the end given to the states. But by then it had largely done its job.

By 1977, when Carter's commission was created, the CMHC program may have, in the natural course of things, been ready to be put out to pasture, for there was probably little more than it could do as a categorical program. It had transformed the landscape of psychiatric care in America. Psychiatric hospitals, particularly state-run institutions, were no longer the dominant vehicle for delivering care to the mentally ill. The mental health profession was no longer exclusively the domain of psychiatrists, and thus of the medical profession; now psychologists, social workers, psychiatric nurses and other mental health professionals shared the task of providing care. The care of the chronically mentally ill that the state hospitals were discharging was the more serious problem, but for centers to service them adequately would require some change.

What is more, in the latter part of the 1970s, as we have seen, the categorical grant program became a phenomenon of the past. As part of an historical movement, the political system was getting ready to yield the responsibility for such efforts to states and local communities, and because of increasing problems with the federal budget there would be fewer dollars to spend on mental health care.

During the later 1960s and early 1970s the CMHC program had been an important force in the development of federal health policy. Before the full effects of the deficits caused by the Vietnam War had taken hold, money was plentiful (by the standards of the 1980s) for such domestic programs, and the centers program as well as other health programs were reasonably well funded, although they never got as much as their advocates said they should get. The CMHC program was sufficiently popular with members of Congress that it was able to pull many other health programs through to enactment along with it, since they were often combined together in an omnibus health bill. But as these programs moved into the next phase, the one in which Congress was writing into the authorizing legislation particulars about how the programs should be administered, and thus telling the managers in the bureaucracy very specifically what they were to do with the money, appropriations were becoming less plentiful and competition for that money between individual health programs became more severe. The mental health program, which did not have the strong economic constituency behind it that other programs had, began to lose strength.

The 1975 amendments to the CMHC program, in addition to becoming more detailed in their directives to the bureaucracy, also added provisions that required new services of centers. All these new elements combined to make greater expectations for the program than could be realized.

Thus, when the Carter mental health commission convened, the feeling was beginning to develop, both in and out of Congress, that the program could no longer serve the public adequately. Furthermore, dissolution of the categorical grant program as a device by which to carry out public policy in the health area was on the horizon, even if the members did not fully realize it. The Carter commission's work and the resulting Mental Health Systems Act nicely set the stage for the changes that Ronald Reagan would propose and be able to carry out. It was typical of what happened to many other categorical health grant programs.

The NHI Effort Fades Away

As 1979 ended, it appeared that a Long-Carter national health insurance bill might actually go to the Senate floor in 1980. The chances were, it seemed, that it would arrive on the floor as the session was going into its final hours. Then the House would have to take it up, but since the measure in the Senate would probably be attached to legislation that had already passed the House, the Carter-Long NHI bill could be approved, and perhaps modified, in conference and then sent off to the White House. Thus, in the helter-skelter activity that invariably accompanied the closing hours of a session, this scenario suggested, Long would be successful, as had been his tradition, of having one of his bills the major piece of legislation to clear Congress just before adjournment.

The brightest days for national health insurance were in March 1980 as the Finance Committee worked further on its measure. In a series of topsy-turvy sessions, the panel wrote a plan that filled the easiest gaps and pushed as much of the cost as possible onto the employer. But in the end the committee was not able to fill enough of the gaps to make the measure politically acceptable, largely because it could not deal with the matter of controlling health care costs.

The Finance bill required employers to provide catastrophic health insurance to full-time employees. Employees, for whom participation would be mandatory unless covered under another program, could be required to pay up to 25 percent of the cost of the insurance premium, with employers paying the rest. Coverage would begin within a month after employment and, if a person was employed at least one year, it would have to continue for ninety days after he or she left the job, or until the person was covered elsewhere. The program was designed to provide coverage to the family unit, not just the individual employee, and dependents would be covered for a year following death, divorce or separation, or until covered by another plan. The standard for the scope of coverage would be Medicare. Employer plans would have to cover hospital costs, physician fees and some nursing and home care. Coverage would start once an employee had paid $3,500 in any one year for medical expenses. Employers would be encouraged to provide other insurance plans that would offer precatastrophic payment for medical care, and expenses under such a program (whether paid for by the insurance company or the employee) would serve to trigger the catastrophic coverage once the $3,500 level of expenses was reached. Employees earning less than $14,000 annually would have a lower catastrophic trigger, as would Medicare beneficiaries.

The Finance Committee's plan in its totality would cost the federal government an estimated $3.2 billion in the first year; the cost to employers would be $6.8 billion and to employees $1.9 billion in higher payroll taxes.

Once the catastrophic plan was tentatively agreed to, the committee set about trying to provide health care for the uninsured poor, but despite its apparent desire to do so, the committee was not able to overcome the formidable task of finding a way to pay for it. Members did spend some time toying with the possibility of increasing taxes on cigarettes and alcohol, but that approach was abandoned before a vote was taken.

During this period, Long was clearly at odds with other members of the Finance Committee, both Republicans and Democrats, in his desire to write a program first and figure out how to pay for it later. Most of his colleagues felt strongly that revenues to pay for a new health care program should be identified first, and the plan tailored to anticipated income.

Also during this period, the economy was unraveling further, President Carter's reelection effort was bogging down; he continued to be preoccupied with the problems of Americans being held hostage in Iran; and it was generally not a time to push for the enactment of new domestic legislation.

As the economy worsened with the warming of both the weather and the presidential campaign, President Carter decided that he should revise his recently released budget to give it a more austere look. This version reduced total federal health spending by $400 million. Many of the cuts were made in programs—such as preventive health care, health maintenance organizations and new ways for training health care personnel—that the Carter administration had been strengthening in recent years in an effort, among other things, to better lay the foundation for national health insurance.

The budget crunch had its effect on the Finance Committee's efforts to write a national health insurance program. Even when it got back to writing its version of the bill in March, there was increasing resistance to going ahead with the task. Bob Dole, the ranking Republican on the panel, wanted to defer further committee action until the Senate had completed work on the budget so the panel would have a firm idea of the overall limitations Congress was likely to adopt.

But Long, persisting, argued that if the committee failed to write a bill, the measure might get brought up on the floor and others would be able to move ahead with their version of national health insurance. Long probably was not concerned about an NHI bill coming to the floor that had not gone through his committee, but he still saw the opportunity for enactment of at least a limited national health insurance program in 1980 and, quite clearly, he wanted to capitalize on it. He was using whatever tactic he could to move the committee ahead. But now the committee's task was being complicated, for when the House and Senate wrote the budget plan for the following year, each committee was charged with making savings, and Long knew that if he did not move ahead with a national health insurance program quickly it would become embroiled in the effort to save money that was looming on the horizon.

As the committee continued its deliberations through the month, the activity became more frenetic. Estimates of the cost of different programs in the billions, sometimes in the hundreds of billions, of dollars were being tossed about. No one had a firm or realistic idea of what the costs would be once the program was enacted, and that was clearly the element that most concerned the members. Even when they spotted creative ways of paying for the program, like raising the tax on tobacco and alcohol, they could not seem to get to the point of adopting a proposal.

By the middle of May the effort of national health insurance had become inextricably intertwined with hospital cost containment in the committee's deliberations, although the latter, most agreed, as a separate piece of legislation, had died with its defeat in the House the previous fall. Although most other members of the committee had lost interest, Long was still, at least for the record, dedicated to the idea. But he, too, soon lost interest, as he returned ever more frequently to Louisiana to campaign for his own reelection.

By the end of May, it was clear that in 1980 there would not be approval of any kind of national health insurance bill, catastrophic or otherwise. The proposal faded away without a whimper.

The panel had been able to agree on a catastrophic health insurance plan and had they come close to completing work on a bill, they probably would have agreed to mandate that employers provide more than catastrophic coverage for their workers. Where they bogged down completely was in providing health insurance for the poor beyond what existed through Medicaid—the cost was just too great.

It takes both the House and the Senate to enact legislation, of course, and during this period there was virtually no activity in the House, although brief hearings were held at one point. With Al Ullman and other leaders of the Ways and Means Committee very cautious—if not opposed—to national health insurance, even to a limited catastrophic plan, any bill passed by the Senate would have had rough going in the

House. On the other hand, the fall legislative session in a presidential election year is very unpredictable, as all—particularly Long—were aware. Had the Finance Committee's bill found its way to the Senate floor and then to the House, momentum would perhaps have developed to send it all the way to the president's desk. Whether that would have happened, we'll never know. What we do know, however, is that once again the task of both filling the gaps in health insurance and controlling health care costs proved too much of an obstacle to be overcome by the Finance Committee.

4
THE REAGAN YEARS AND BEYOND

With the election of Ronald Reagan the possibility of immediate enactment of a national health insurance program in any form similar to Kennedy's original Health Security Act, or even to Carter's 1979 national health plan, faded entirely from the national agenda. Reagan was firmly against anything called national health insurance, equating any such program with socialized medicine. And the support for him in Congress solidified that view into national policy.

Whether national health insurance would resurface in the future as a political possibility would depend on the exigencies of American politics. If Reagan were replaced in 1985 by a Democratic president, particularly one who called himself a liberal, national health insurance would likely rise up again. It was a point of irony that as Reagan and Congress pared away during Reagan's term at the benefits available under Medicare and Medicaid as well as reducing federal support for other kinds of health programs, they were dissolving the glue that was a principal reason national health insurance had not moved along further. With Medicare and Medicaid and private insurance, most Americans (all but approximately 20 million) were pretty well covered for health costs—not ideally, but pretty well—and thus there was no driving, large constituency for national health insurance. With the changes made in federal support for health during the Reagan era, that complacency could dissolve, and the constituency for NHI might be galvanized sufficiently to push through a substantial new program, once Reagan left office.

But that would require a significant change in the body politic. In the meantime, during the early 1980s, there was little chance for serious congressional consideration of national health insurance; in fact, during the 97th Congress from 1981 to 1982, Kennedy did not reintroduce either of his NHI bills—neither the 1971 Health Security Act nor the 1979 Health Care for All Americans Act, and no one else made an issue of national health insurance. Instead, the talk in the Reagan era was about making the health care marketplace more competitive.

Competition Becomes the Vogue

Competition, of course, is an all-encompassing term. The primary benefit of more competition in the health arena, according to Reagan's health policy-makers, would be to dampen health care inflation. Achieving more competition, however, would require breaking down the triangle of physician, patient and insurance company that had so long dominated and creating an environment providing incentives to those who received health care to make decisions based, in part at least, on what it would cost.

In some ways, although not in prices for services, there had always been a substantial amount of competition in the health care sector. There was competition among students to gain acceptance to medical school, and competition among doctors to get patients and to keep them. There was also competition to produce new and better equipment and technical apparatus.

Competition in health services initially did not mean cut-rate surgery and price wars. Many people when they talked about stimulating competition in the health care marketplace meant eliminating much, if not all, federal regulation, such as the Health Planning Act, that supposedly encumbered the health care industry. Others saw the need for a greater variety of insurance plans, offering the consumer more choice. But by mid-1983 competition over prices charged for services was becoming a factor in health care delivery in some instances; the health care market was beginning to change significantly.

The concept of improving competition in the health care marketplace was not original with the Reagan administration—some legislators had been talking about it since the mid-1970s—but with Reagan's election it became, initially, the only game in town.

Numerous proposals were introduced in the late 1970s and early 1980s designed to stimulate competition in the health care sector. Essentially, competition proposals addressed four basic deficiencies in the existing system. The first was the problem of excessive tax deductions. Another was an insurance system that insulated consumers from the actual cost of health care. Third was the fee-for-service system that most policy-makers felt encouraged physicians to increase both the quantity and price of their services so as to increase their income. The fourth was the system by which hospitals were paid for their services—essentially reimbursements for costs, which gave the hospital an incentive to increase expenditures.

One of the most forceful and certainly the most active exponents of these competition proposals was Alain Enthoven, an economics professor at Stanford University who in 1977 produced for Joseph Califano, Carter's first secretary of Health, Education and Welfare, a national health insurance plan. Enthoven's plan, although originally written for Califano, served as the touchstone for most competition plans; it was the one all others kept coming back to, and Enthoven during the latter 1970s spent much time traveling between Palo Alto, California, and Washington to push his ideas.

Enthoven argued that existing federal policies that thwarted competition in the health care marketplace should be replaced with ones that stimulated competition. He wanted employers to offer several types of health insurance plans and to contribute the same amount to each one, regardless of what they cost—the employee would have to pay the difference if his plan cost more than the allowable amount. He also wanted to organize doctors into competing economic units, such as health maintenance organizations, although he called also for radical changes in the federal health maintenance organization program. That law, he said, treated HMOs unfairly by placing costly burdens on them that were not imposed on their competitors—the physicians who charged a fee for a service. A third element of the Enthoven plan established a uniform set of rules for health insurance plans covering benefits and premiums among other features.

The proposals of others differed in degree and style as to how they sought to correct the shortcomings in the health care system. The matter of excessive tax deductions would be handled in one of several ways, but they all boiled down to placing a limit on the amount an employer could pay for an employee's health care; anything over that cap would become taxable income to the employee. Some proposals, as an encouragement to employees to choose less-expensive plans, allowed them to keep the difference between the cap and the cost of the plan they chose as nontaxable income. Some proposals would also eliminate the medical deduction for the individual taxpayer or reduce the impact of it. These changes would remove at least some of the insulation that protected the patient from the cost of health care.

Other proposals adopted the Enthoven principle that required employers to offer employees a choice of several health insurance plans, and often one of those choices had to be an HMO. In order for an insurance plan to qualify, it usually would have to meet certain requirements, such as providing minimum benefits, specifying the size of the family unit it would cover, making sure that coverage continued after employment until additional coverage became effective and requiring insurance for catastrophic health care costs. By forcing competition among plans, physicians and hospitals, it was expected, would hold down costs in order to make their services more attractive.

Some bills proposed converting the Medicare and Medicaid programs, at least in part, into voucher systems, whereby the beneficiaries could receive a specific payment with which they could purchase health insurance. This would, it was believed, remove the monopoly of Medicare and Medicaid as payers of health care costs for the aged and poor and in so doing help hold down costs.

Two of the key players in developing health policy in Ronald Reagan's administration—Richard Schweiker, the president's first secretary of the Department of Health and Human Services, and David Stockman, director of the Office of Management and Budget—had as members of Congress already strongly pushed the competition concept. Stockman in 1980 as a representative proposed, along with his colleague, Richard

Gephardt, the Missouri Democrat who had sponsored the antihospital cost-containment amendment in the House in 1979, legislation that sought through a number of financial incentives to urge consumers to seek out the best buy in insurance. Like other competition proposals, it set a limit on the amount an employer could contribute to an employee's health insurance without the employee having more taxable income, and it provided tax credits to those who chose to reduce significantly their spending for health insurance. Medicare and Medicaid beneficiaries would be given the dollars, in the form of vouchers, with which to purchase health insurance, if they chose. But the Stockman bill went beyond most competition proposals and proposed eliminating a number of regulatory programs, such as the Health Planning Act, which the sponsors argued thwarted competition. In short, it sought to remove the federal government from directly financing and regulating health services. For Stockman, so determined to remove the federal government from the health care sector, the measure required a good deal of federal regulation by qualifying health insurance plans.

Schweiker, like Stockman, was no novice to health issues when he became part of the Reagan government in January 1981. Before coming to the job of HHS secretary, he had spent twenty years in Congress, the last twelve as a senator from Pennsylvania, where he had served as a principal in the development of health programs, although as a Republican and thus a member during those years of the Senate's minority party. Schweiker had been, for several years before he retired from the Senate in early 1981, the ranking Republican on both the health subcommittee of the Labor and Human Resources Committee, which was responsible for all health legislation supporting specialized or categorical programs, and on the subcommittee of the Appropriations Committee that was responsible each year for writing the money bill for the Department of Health and Human Services.

As a senator in 1979, Schweiker sponsored legislation that would have required employers to offer employees at least three health insurance programs, one of which would have to be a prepaid plan. A typical provision of the procompetition bills, it, of course, would be direct government interference, for it set a mandated federal requirement for those insurance programs. What is more, the federal government would have to establish a mechanism to qualify those plans, thus creating more government apparatus. Under Schweiker's proposal, like Stockman's, the different plans were expected to compete with each other to attract purchasers. Since the employer was limited in what he could pay on behalf of the employee and since employees who chose a plan less costly than the established target price could get the difference in tax-free income, health insurance plans would strive to reduce costs while keeping benefits up. To be able to hold down price increases in the cost of policies the companies would have to work to keep hospitals and physicians from raising their prices.

A principal issue in all competition proposals has been tax deductions for expenses related to the delivery and support of health care.

One of the favorite ways the American government has of dealing with an issue is through the tax code. Taxes may be anathema to most people, but one's ability to take advantage of a tax exemption becomes a matter of pride and prestige. Congress and the administration have together fiddled with the tax code over the years to the extent that in 1983 the federal government made a $23.7-billion investment in the nation's health care system. By 1987 without any changes in the law that investment would climb to $38 billion.[151]

The investment was the result of taxes that did not flow to the Treasury because of exemptions permitted for medical care and related expenditures. And as usual those who got the most advantages from these exemptions were the very rich, while those who received almost no advantage were the poor.

Tax exemptions for health take several forms. Employers are allowed to deduct what they spend on health care for their employees—either through the purchase of insurance or in payment for direct care—from taxable income of the business because it is considered an expense of doing business. Although the money deducted becomes taxable income to someone else—the insurance company or the provider of health care, if not nonprofit and thus tax exempt—it does not become taxable income to the principal beneficiary, the employee.

In a similar way, individual taxpayers are allowed to deduct certain medical expenses from their income taxes—in 1983 those that exceeded 5 percent of adjusted gross income. Contributions to charities that deliver or otherwise support health services, research and training could also be taken as a tax deduction.

One further deduction was permitted in 1983—under certain circumstances hospitals and other health care facilities might have access to revenue raised from the sale of bonds the interest for which was tax exempt, a device that tended to encourage the construction of new hospitals and thus often the creation of unneeded hospital beds.

Tax deductions for health care costs began in 1942 when taxes on incomes were substantially increased and the base broadened to help finance the war. In order to compensate for this change, the deduction for those with high medical costs was also increased on the grounds that extraordinary medical expenses reduced one's ability to pay income taxes. It was, in addition, a way of providing more income to workers whose wages could not be raised because of a wartime freeze.

Tax exemptions generally are rationalized on the grounds that money freed from taxation is to be used in certain beneficial ways. In the health area, the assumption is that people will get better health care.

In 1983, if workers had had to pay income tax on the amount employers paid in their behalf for health insurance, the federal government would have gotten $18.1 billion in additional revenues. If people in filing their tax returns had not been allowed to deduct any of their health care costs, tax revenues would have increased by $4.2 billion. Deductions in 1983 to charities for health purposes amounted to a loss of $1.1 billion in federal revenues, while the loss that year to the federal government because of the sale of tax-exempt bonds was $250 million.[152]

It is difficult to tell to what extent and how this investment through the tax code affects the nation's health care system, but there is no doubt the $24-billion—and rising—annual investment has an impact. In fact, the federal government's investment in health through the tax system is the second-largest federal investment in health, ranking only behind that made through the Medicare program.

One way the influence of this investment is felt is that employers are encouraged to purchase more, rather than less, health insurance for their employees, since it is a way of providing additional benefits without those benefits becoming taxable income to the worker and the employer does not have to pay social security tax. And those who have extraordinary health care coverage are likely to use the services they pay for because the care will cost them little or nothing.

But the benefits flow from this exemption unequally. The best rates for health insurance and usually the best policies go to those who purchase it as a member of a large group. If one is self-employed, or employed by a small firm, the rates are likely to be high and the benefits not as good. Thus, many people because of the way they earn their living are effectively barred from the best health care insurance and thus, perhaps, the best in health care.

Furthermore, tax savings to individuals for deductions for the cost of medical care are of a much greater advantage to people with high incomes than to those with low incomes. As a 1980 study of the Congressional Budget Office pointed out, "For affluent households, who are the prime beneficiaries of the deduction, it can provide generous subsidies for plastic surgery, trips to warm climates and other types of elective care."[153]

The CBO report contended that if the medical deduction were repealed, some people with high incomes might pay as much as $5,000 in additional taxes (and some of the very wealthy with high medical expenses might even pay much more) while those with low incomes would pay very little, if anything, more. But as a practical matter, very few low-income persons itemized deductions on their income tax return and thus did not take advantage of this loophole. Roughly 72 percent of all taxpayers do not itemize deductions.

If all tax deductions for health care and related expenditures were eliminated, people would be more cautious about how they spent their health care dollars. The change would have a limited impact on the use of insurance, except that its costs would no longer be deductible, for policies providing elegant coverage would still be available. If the expense were not deductible people would think more seriously about whether the health care they purchased was really necessary because the portion of the cost not covered by insurance would be fully taxed. Removing tax exemptions is an important step in bringing the patient squarely into the decision-making process.

What is more, such a change, if the entire exemption were removed, would provide a $24-billion increase in federal tax revenues.

Like much of federal health policy, elements of the tax code contradict other established principles. One of the central issues in the general debate over the proper federal role in paying for health care services is the extent to which it is desirable to have people pay for some of their health care so they will be aware of the cost, or whether it is better to have no barriers to health care services so that they will seek care when they need it and thus hopefully prevent the need for more expensive treatment at a later date. Most people involved in making or analyzing health policy now take the position that health insurance coverage should involve both deductibles (the patient paying front-end costs, such as the first day of hospitalization) and copayments (paying a portion of all costs, such as 20 percent), at least up to a specified maximum amount, where catastrophic coverage might take over.

The exemptions in the tax code have an impact on this debate because the pressure on employers is to provide more and more comprehensive health care coverage for their workers, while the employees make smaller and smaller payments for the actual services rendered.

It is pressure that organized labor, particularly, during the 1960s and 1970s increasingly exerted on management, but also increasingly over the objection of management. It has been primarily because of management's resistance that labor has pushed for enactment of national health insurance. Labor wanted to get health care costs off the bargaining table.

Because deductions are a permanent part of the tax code, the revenue losses they create are not subject to regular congressional review. Thus, this form of subsidization of the health care system is rarely taken into account by Congress when considering health proposals. CBO Director Alice Rivlin in testimony before a joint hearing of the House Ways and Means and Budget committees in July 1979 argued that tax incentives for health insurance "are among the most important ways the federal government influences health care in the United States."[154] And yet, they have been paid, for the most part, the least attention by those who make federal health policy.

One change was made in 1982. When Congress enacted that year's tax bill, it reduced the exemptions that individual taxpayers can claim for health care costs. The change was expected to cut $272 million from the health care tax expenditure in 1983, rising to a saving of nearly $2 billion by 1987. At an early stage in its deliberations, the Finance Committee considered placing a cap on the amount employers could contribute to employee health care costs, but business, labor and health insurance companies all lobbied against it and the panel shifted to the path of least resistance. President Reagan in 1983 again proposed a limit on the amount an employer could contribute to an employee's health insurance, and once again the opposition increased.

The tax benefit for health expenditures, when it was created during World War II, was aimed primarily at helping the working man, members of organized labor, and today health benefits, as noted, are still a major item in labor-management contracts. Labor, of course, has been one of the major backers of a comprehensive national health program, but short of enactment of a full-fledged national health insurance program to take over where health insurance programs sponsored by the employer would leave off, labor has been reluctant to make incremental changes in existing health policy, such as changes in the tax laws, that might lead to a more rational system. If the tax exclusion were eliminated, except for those who are well paid and members of unions like the United Auto Workers that have aggressively pursued health benefits in their bargaining contracts, the impact for most workers would be small. But it was not a benefit, in the general sense of things, that labor leaders could give up without getting something in return. In the meantime, the big winners from this provision in the tax laws were, once again, the very rich who got a bonus they did not really need.

There were many who objected to the competition proposals for a variety of reasons. The tax cap, a device to cut down on the loss of revenues to the Treasury, was seen by some as unworkable. Healthy people would choose the cheaper plans so as to get the extra cash while high-risk people would choose the insurance plan with the best benefits, sending the cost of those programs even higher.

Proposals mandating that employees be given the opportunity to choose among several competing health insurance plans would hurt, some suggested, those employers who used the leverage provided by large purchases of insurance to bargain for lower rates and of others who self-insured, or set aside funds within the business to cover health care costs rather than purchasing insurance from a commercial company.

But mostly, the plans were criticized for relieving government of the responsibility to assure that everyone had available a minimum level of health care and for asking the consumer to make sophisticated decisions about the purchase of health insurance and protection of their own well-being that many thought they were not capable of making.

Karen Davis, deputy HHS assistant secretary for Planning and Evaluation for Health in the Carter administration, was one of the more persistent critics who argued for going slow on competition. In hearings before the House Ways and Means Committee early in 1980, Davis stressed that competition could not be "an end in itself" and that procompetitive proposals should be examined to "be sure they conform with other social goals." She was particularly concerned that enhancing competition by requiring patients to pay more from their own pockets for their health care would result in the poor getting less health care than they needed. She also argued that there was "little evidence" to indicate the procompetition proposals could "provide substantial immediate relief from health care inflation—or that competitive approaches can effect more than marginal changes in the health care system."[155]

The factors that impeded competition and its potential for containing costs, Davis later told the Senate Finance Committee, "are deeply ingrained in the health care system." One of the principal reasons the health care industry would not respond to rational competitive incentives, she argued, was that the decisions were all made by physicians.[156]

CBO's Rivlin, testifying before the House Ways and Means Committee, said that competition plans might, within five years, shave as much as $8 billion from the national health care bill while increasing federal revenues by a possible $6 billion. But, she argued, procompetition legislation was not a substitute for hospital cost containment or for comprehensive health insurance proposals, although it would complement both efforts.[157]

Patricia Harris, Califano's successor as secretary of the Department of Health and Human Services, in a June 1980 speech said that competition proposals that made the consumer pay more through increased copayments and higher deductibles would "place a disproportionately heavy burden on those least able to pay for health services," and, she added, "I do not believe that in seeking to create a more efficient and more competitive health care system we ought to place the burden of cost containment" on the poor. "It is one thing to ask a patient to pay a few dollars more before insurance steps in," Harris said, "and quite another to ask that of the poor or even the moderate income working families already struggling to make ends meet."[158]

There were other problems with the competition proposals besides the fact they would undermine, if not do away with, the established ethic that government had a responsibility to insure everyone with a minimum level of health care. The competition concept also undermined certain established principles for the health care community (the patient aside) that have tended to protect the leaders in the industry from economic hardship.

Competition in the traditional free market sense means that new business can enter the field freely, and that businesses can go bankrupt if they cannot earn enough money to pay their bills. This is the way the free market has of dealing with excessive investment. The possibility of health care facilities, and particularly hospitals, going bankrupt is anathema to most communities and thus to the people who govern them. This is especially true of public hospitals serving the poor, usually in inner cities. During the late Carter years several efforts were made by the federal government to provide financial support, through special Medicare-Medicaid reimbursement schemes and other devices, to save several nearly bankrupt hospitals in New York City. Those hospitals were rescued for the moment, but by mid-1983 they were again threatened as unemployed workers without health insurance turned to them for free care.

Likewise, entry into the industry is not all that simple. Take hospitals again. The health planning act required that health planning agencies give permission for a new hospital to start up, or even to expand to include new services or more beds. Even without the planning act there are barriers—a principal one being accreditation, a procedure devised by and under the aegis of the medical care industry itself. Accreditation is necessary before a hospital can, in most cases, receive reimbursements from insurance companies and the federal government. Physicians, too, must pass certain exams before they can be licensed to practice independently, although for most this has not been a difficult barrier. The whole procedure of accrediting facilities and individuals has, in fact, provided a major argument as to why the federal government should not touch the matter.

Few who advocated competition proposals were willing to allow the health care market to operate totally unfettered. Stockman came the closest—he clearly believed it was necessary to allow hospitals to go bankrupt; to go out of business because they could not earn enough to pay their bills—as a device to clear out of the way inefficient systems. But other aspects of his plan called for government regulation, such as establishing requirements for health care plans.

Stockman saw a need, as others had, to set limits on the value of health care services being made available to the poor and the elderly, through transfers of wealth and resources using the tax system. But Stockman wanted to set limits on these transfers by converting federal aid to the poor and elderly into vouchers with a specific monetary value, vouchers that they would use to purchase insurance in the private market. In this way, the Medicare and Medicaid programs would ultimately be done away with. That the Medicare or Medicaid beneficiary would have to deal in the marketplace like everyone else was a threatening idea to Democratic liberals.

The thought of changing the way the health care market operated probably never would have arisen if health prices had remained moderate, but since they did not, policy-makers searched for a device to bring down that inflation, and, after other approaches either failed or were rejected, they found competition. Most Democratic liberals saw it simply as a smoke screen to cover over the dismantlement, without any replacement, of Medicare and Medicaid. Thus, the issue really became what was the commitment made by the United States government when it adopted those programs. It was perhaps an irrelevant controversy, since such commitments are never irrevocable. But the most captivating point was that, no matter who proposed the plan, or what the elements were, it always required some regulation by the federal government. There was no way of getting around it, unless all pretense at achieving some degree of fairness was abandoned. And very few, if any, were prepared to do that.

Reagan's Health Policy Agenda

With Ronald Reagan in the White House in January 1981, it was thought that the new administration would soon be coming forward with its procompetition health care plan. But like the Carter administration and its national health insurance plan, the Reagan administration took longer than expected. And before he got to work on such a plan, the new president first started cutting back on all types of federal health spending. He accomplished this by using a device called reconciliation that had been put into the Budget Control and Impoundment Act of 1974—that bill created and enacted by a Democratic Congress to help it thwart the budget policies of a Republican president of whom it did not approve. It was a device that had lain dormant until 1980 when President Carter used it, also to trim domestic spending as a way of cutting the deficit.

Reconciliation was designed to be used by Congress each fall to help it bring its work of the session into line with the budget plan that it had adopted the previous spring. That plan was to serve as the blueprint for committees as they went about writing appropriations bills providing money to be spent in the upcoming fiscal year, making new expenditures through entitlement programs (which circumvented the appropriations process), and passing legislation to raise revenues. If, as Congress approached the start of the new fiscal year on the first of October, the 1974 budget act said, it found expenditures and revenues were not in line with the budget plan, then, through a reconciliation bill, Congress would issue directives to itself to pare back spending in one or more appropriation acts or in entitlement legislation, such as the Medicare and Medicaid programs, or raise additional revenues, or accept a larger debt. It was, conceptually, a good technique, but the original concept would be redesigned.

While President Carter was the first to use the budget reconciliation device, President Reagan turned it into a major instrument of policy-making, and in so doing was able to cut big chunks out of the federal government's health bill. In 1981, he got Congress to enact a reconciliation bill as the first order of the year's business, turning it into a major device to restructure spending priorities as opposed to being merely an end-of-the-year adjustment technique. In the first spring of his presidency, Reagan won enactment of proposals as part of an omnibus reconciliation bill making substantial changes in Medicare and Medicaid as well as other federal health programs. In effect, he told Congress, "Here is what I want to do. It's all here in one bill and all you have to do is enact it." And with the help of a Senate dominated by Republicans (for the first time since 1954) and a House dominated by a coalition of

Republicans and conservative Democrats, Reagan was able to get much of his package enacted. In his second year in office, Reagan was able to win more changes in the way the Medicare program operated, and as part of the 1983 social security reform legislation he got Congress to agree to a plan placing limits on what Medicare would pay for hospital services.

These changes in federal health policy were, in reality, the culmination of an evolutionary process that had been going on for about ten years—ever since Richard Nixon after the midterm election of 1970 started articulating the new direction he would follow.

Nixon, as we saw, wanted to cut back the federal investment for health, get away from involvement in a lot of specialized health programs and substitute instead a national health insurance program. But he really made only modest advancements toward his goals. His cutbacks were thwarted by Congress and his national health insurance plan disappeared about the time he was forced from office. But President Ford, in his own way, continued the effort and it was under his presidency that health block grants were first aggressively proposed. Although that idea was rejected by the Democratic Congress, there was then, as we saw, considerable sympathy for it. Under Ford, too, the decision was essentially made to get the federal government out of the business of paying for the education of physicians, since doctor shortages were about to become a thing of the past. It was also during the Ford era that Senator Talmadge first developed his Medicare-Medicaid reform bill that laid the groundwork for the 1983 legislation setting limits on Medicare hospital payments.

During Carter's four years in office, the effort to extract the federal government from supporting the training of physicians was continued, and while the block grants were not again offered, some consolidation and redirection was accomplished, as with mental health services.

Reagan's 1981 reconciliation bill proposed converting most specialized or categorical health programs into block grants and making a number of changes in the Medicare and Medicaid programs that would trim their costs. The legislation as finally passed did not go as far as he wanted, but it set the direction of federal health policy for the next several years.

As enacted, the legislation converted existing categorical health grant programs into four health block grants: preventive health services; alcohol, drug abuse and mental health; primary care; and maternal and child health. Under this scheme, the federal government would hand over each year a chunk of money to each of the states to operate health programs that had been lumped together into the block grant. Federal directives and regulations were minimized, giving states more freedom in how they spent the money, and the total amount of federal dollars invested in these programs was reduced.

The block grants had their impact on the amount spent by the federal government. In fiscal 1981, the year Carter left office, the combined appropriations for the health programs put into the block grants was $1.4 billion. In fiscal 1982 it was $1.1 billion, a drop of 21.8 percent. The decline had started with Carter's request to rescind part of the fiscal 1981 budget enacted in the fall of 1980 (which Reagan soon after he entered office got Congress to amend, making even further reductions). That year's budget for this group of programs carried a 7.6 percent reduction over the fiscal 1980 funding of $1.5 billion.[159]

The changes initially proposed by the Reagan government for Medicare largely affected reimbursements to hospitals. Congress went this one better by raising the amount of the deductible Medicare beneficiaries would have to pay at the beginning of a hospital stay, and increased the deductible for physician services. The sum total of the changes was to mean higher health costs for Medicare beneficiaries.

Changes in Medicaid enacted as part of the 1981 bill reduced the federal government's share of Medicaid costs over the following three years by an estimated 3 percent in the first year and 4.5 percent in the third—less than the flat 5 percent cap on increased expenditures the administration had wanted. The changes also gave states, which were feeling the pressure of rising Medicaid costs just as acutely as the federal government, substantial discretion over services that would be provided to some Medicaid beneficiaries and over how they paid for services. The changes had the desired effect. Carolyne Davis, Reagan's administrator of the Medicare and Medicaid programs, was able to report in 1983 that the changes two years earlier reduced Medicaid spending by 9.5 percent a year in 1983 and 1984, down from 15 percent in fiscal 1980.[160] What had happened, though, was that the cost of care was, at least to some degree, being shifted to the Medicaid beneficiary. A 1982 study by the Urban Institute reported that "states are actively constraining Medicaid benefits and payments."[161]

The fact that the reconciliation bill was less sweeping with regard to its health block grants than originally proposed by the president, while most of its other provisions were very much in line with what the White House wanted, was viewed by many as a victory, and a substantial accomplishment, for Henry Waxman, the chairman of the House Commerce health subcommittee. Waxman had dealt with Reagan before—when he was chairman of a similar panel in the California legislature while Reagan was governor. Now he was taking on Reagan again. In conference with the Senate over differing versions of the bill, Waxman was able to preserve the House position that parsed many of the categorical health grant programs into four different block grants rather than lumping them all together in one. And he was able to preserve, as well, at least in some cases, much of the individual integrity of the programs. This would be important if he wanted to rebuild them as separate programs at a later date, perhaps under a different administration. Waxman was also able to thwart putting as severe a limit on additional federal Medicaid expenses each year as Reagan had wanted. After that accomplishment Waxman was hailed by many as a coming power in the House.

If within the confines of the Congress-Reagan battle of 1981 Waxman was a winner, in the larger context of the overall shift in federal health policy and his efforts to prevent that, he was a loser, for with the enactment of the 1981 reconciliation bill, some very significant changes had been made in health policy.

Waxman in a 1983 interview obviously was taking pride in his 1981 accomplishment, but at the same time he was unable to describe what he wanted federal health policy to look like, beyond acknowledging that there were many issues that needed to be studied. He saw his job during these Reagan years as a holding action, preserving as much as possible the integrity of the old-time programs. He had not yet looked to the future, he said, to see how a new and more productive and constructive system might be built.

Reagan returned in 1982 to propose more changes, and in that year's omnibus tax bill, Medicare costs were trimmed by $12 billion over the next three years. Limits were placed on reimbursements to hospitals for ancillary services—almost everything beyond bed, board and nursing care—and on the amount a hospital's total reimbursements through Medicare could rise each year. The tax bill also provided that Medicare would pay only for the health care costs of beneficiaries who continued to work—and thus had access through employment to private health insurance policies—if those private policies would not pay for services covered by Medicare. Thus, in another way, more of the burden of the cost of health care was shifted to employers.

Initially Reagan administration policy-makers thought the problem of rising health care costs could be solved by developing a procompetition health care plan. But by mid-1982 work on the plan was seriously bogged down. There were two problems: The administration was beleaguered by more serious issues, primarily the huge budget deficit, and the White House clearly did not want to put forward a health care proposal that would interfere with efforts of the moment to get its tax bill passed.

By January 1983, however, the administration was ready to make its proposal public, but competition in the forms described earlier by Enthoven, Stockman and Schweiker, while included, would not provide the main ingredient. Instead, the new Reagan initiative attempted to cut back on inflation in the Medicare program by putting a cap on what the federal government would pay for hospital services and by requiring beneficiaries to pay more of the cost of hospitalization. But under the Reagan plan there was to be a limit to what beneficiaries would pay—

catastrophic coverage would be provided. After an elderly person had spent about $1,500 of his own money, all remaining costs would be covered.

As originally designed, the Medicare and Medicaid programs reimbursed hospitals for the cost of treating beneficiaries—costs that could vary, sometimes dramatically, from one area of the country to another. Under the new system proposed by the Reagan administration, the federal government would say how much it would pay for a hospital for each type of treatment—repairing a broken hip, removing a kidney stone, or whatever. If the hospital's actual cost was less than what Medicare paid, the facility could keep the difference. If it was more, it would have to absorb the loss.

Whether it was argued that prospective reimbursement was, in a sense, another form of government regulation, and thus a cardinal sin in the Reagan government's lexicon, or simply a matter of the federal government exercising its responsibilities as a prudent buyer, the president really had no other choice if he wanted to stop the hemorrhaging of the Medicare trust fund.

The plan was a major step in an effort to derail the pell-mell drive toward bankruptcy of the Medicare hospital trust fund, which in mid-1983 was expected to occur by the end of the decade, if not earlier, but it would not do the job alone. In its first year, as incorporated with some changes into the social security legislation passed by Congress in the spring of 1983, the full effects of the plan would not be felt until the end of a three-year phase-in period. Nevertheless, it set the stage for more sweeping changes to the Medicare program later on; a breach had been made in the reimbursement scheme, and that was very important. Although it applied only to Medicare reimbursements and not to all hospital costs, the legislation capitalized on the experience of Carter's hospital cost-containment effort—and many of those inside Congress and out who had opposed that program became supporters of the 1983 effort. In part, they were closer to desperation and saw calamity on the horizon; in part, the new administration had more support for its proposal and the entire undertaking was carried out in a less confrontational environment.

Some of the principles proposed by the advocates of competition did appear in the 1983 Reagan plan. It proposed limiting (at $175 for a family) the amount an employer could pay each month toward an employee's health insurance without the worker's having to pay tax on the payment as if it were income. Furthermore, Medicare beneficiaries would be offered vouchers with which they could purchase private health insurance. This feature built upon a provision enacted by Congress in 1982 making it easy for Medicare beneficiaries to join health maintenance organizations and making it attractive for HMOs to go after this market. The HMO would be paid an amount equal to 95 percent of the average cost of treating an elderly person in that particular area. Although the elderly had been able to swap traditional coverage for HMO coverage ever since the HMO program had been enacted in 1973, there had been little inducement for the HMO to recruit beneficiaries because they were reimbursed for the actual cost of providing care. With enactment of the 1982 law, HMOs could now gamble that they could make money on the elderly by being paid a flat fee by Medicare, and if it cost them less to treat the person they could keep the difference.

The changes made in federal health policy generally, and primarily in the Medicare and Medicaid programs, during the first two and a half years of the Reagan presidency, particularly in light of the record of the previous decade, were remarkable. But, as noted, they capitalized on momentum developed during that decade. Nevertheless, administration officials who had charge of formulating and executing that policy took great pride in these accomplishments. HHS Assistant Secretary for Planning and Evaluation Robert Rubin, a physician, and OMB Executive Associate Director for Budget and Legislation Donald Moran, as well as professional staff members for GOP senators in key health policy spots, in interviews in mid-1983 gave most of the credit to the administration. They particularly took pride in the rapidity with which Congress adopted, as part of the 1983 omnibus social security amendments, the caps on what Medicare would pay for hospital care. But enactment of this legislation was not surprising. Congress, in fact, in 1982 had directed the administration to develop such a proposal and, as noted, by 1983 everyone, including the hospital lobby, was eager to go along with the measure as a way of forestalling more stringent legislation, say along the lines of Jimmy Carter's hospital cost-containment proposal.

Indeed, by mid-1983 there were signs that hospital costs, the most intransigent aspect of inflation in the health care arena, were moderating. Employers by then had become very concerned about the rising cost of health care in their fringe-benefit packages and they were putting pressure on both employees and insurance companies to reduce these costs by giving priority to outpatient care over inpatient care, foregoing elective surgery and taking other cost-saving steps. According to the American Hospital Association, hospital inflation continued to moderate during the first quarter of 1983, and for the year ending that March the rate was 12.9 percent, down from 18 percent for the comparable period a year earlier. That new, lower rate was about where hospital inflation had been when the House in 1979 had rejected President Carter's hospital cost-containment proposal. A major argument in support of that rejection had been that hospital inflation was then about the same as inflation in the economy generally. By the spring of 1983, however, overall inflation had dropped to 3.5 percent.

Don Moran saw all this as clear evidence that the market was beginning to work in a more conventional manner, and he was right. He also suggested that the process would continue, thus mitigating the need for radical federal intervention.

But others saw the need for such intervention on the horizon, and they suggested that it would come after the 1984 election, during what they expected would be Ronald Reagan's second term in the White House. David Winston, a former aide to Richard Schweiker both when he was in the Senate and at the Department of Health and Human Services, and who continued to counsel the administration although no longer a federal employee, in a 1983 interview said he saw a crisis ahead as the Medicare trust fund came closer to bankruptcy. He anticipated that the administration would eventually have to support a cap on all hospital costs as the only way of putting a meaningful damper on inflation in that area. Moran, however, saw the options differently—basically as a choice between raising the Medicare payroll tax and reducing the benefits, and he thought the likelihood was that benefits would be reduced.

Although not part of the plan to hold down the rise in Medicare and Medicaid costs, prevention of illness for the Reagan administration was an important part of its health strategy, just as it had been for its predecessor. But primary responsibility for prevention, the new government said, like responsibility for all other health efforts, was to be vested in state and local governments. The federal government's financial support, under the Reagan plan, for immunization programs would be cut back. That policy involved risks, but how great the risks were depended upon how the possible adverse consequences were valued.

Plague or big epidemics were unlikely. What was likely was that hundreds, perhaps thousands, of children would catch measles, mumps or some other childhood disease and live their lives out with impairments that could have easily been prevented. To keep the federally supported immunization programs at their peak would cost perhaps another $5 million—"a few rounds of ammunition," as one state health officer described it. The issue was, thus, a matter of priorities.

Richard Schweiker, President Reagan's first secretary of Health and Human Services, said over and over again that preventive health was at the top of the list of priorities in the Reagan government's health plan. He also argued that reductions in federal spending for prevention were being picked up by the states and, what is more, some of that reduction, like fewer dollars for immunization, was justified because the goals had been met—that is, immunization of 90 percent or more had been achieved; acceleration was no longer necessary, only maintenance to make sure new youngsters were immunized.

The national immunization system had been considerably strengthened in the immediately preceding years and thus was not likely to fall apart; the health of the population was not in serious jeopardy. There would not be any "rampant outbreaks," state officials conceded, but there would most likely be pockets of disease that could affect hundreds of children, some of whom might be permanently damaged. These tragedies were entirely preventable, and thus should be prevented.

The history of the ups and downs of federal support for immunization appeared to prove this point. As a result in an earlier cut in federal funding for immunization programs, between 1968 and 1970 there was a 30 percent reduction in immunization against measles. Between 1970 and 1971 there was a substantial increase in the incidence of measles. By 1976, federal support for measles had been cut in half, to $2 million, over the 1972 level, and by 1977 the incidence of measles had risen 200 percent over the 1972 level. Federal support for immunization was increased in 1977 and very quickly the incidence of measles dropped. By 1982, measles were a rarity, but they had not been wiped out, as has smallpox, and by the end of the year minor measles epidemics were appearing in certain parts of the country.

Caring for children who are damaged by measles can be very expensive. Over the course of the person's life the cost can be as much as $1 million. The nation in 1982 was spending about $250 million a year—or eight times the federal immunization budget—caring for children born with disabilities resulting from measles. In 1964, a rubella epidemic injured 25,000 children, and the special care they would require for the rest of their lives would run to perhaps $2 billion.

Medicare's Future

At best, the changes to Medicare being proposed by the Reagan government and made by Congress were only setting the stage for even more sweeping changes that would have to be made at a later time.

Medicare is the flagship in the United States health care apparatus, both public and private, and only when the administration and Congress choose to deal with this program head on, rather than just tinkering with it by scaling back benefits, increasing cost sharing or laying caps on what the program will pay providers, will the first significant step be taken to really solving the nation's health care problems.

Medicare is the flagship because it is the payer of health services for the largest single portion of the nation's population. In 1983 it served as the primary source for financing health care for 30 million Americans. Although that was only 14 percent of the 1983 population, it included the most vulnerable portion of all Americans—the elderly (26 million) and the disabled (4 million). While paying for a substantial portion of the cost of care for this group, Medicare was the biggest single source of revenue for hospitals—35 percent—and of the entire health care economy it provided about 17 percent of the income.[162] In this regard, it set the standards for quality of care, the extent of care, and innovations.

While Medicare may pay only 45 percent of the elderly's health care costs, this figure is deceiving. Except for the cost of one hospital day, Medicare in early 1983 paid for sixty days of hospital care in each illness, and it paid a portion of the costs of hospitalization beyond sixty days. Furthermore, it paid 80 percent of an amount that it set for physician and outpatient care, although beneficiaries had to pay a premium of about $140 a year to get this extra insurance. If the actual cost of the service was more than allowed under Medicare, the patient paid for the difference, as well as the standard 20 percent. But often much if not all of this amount was paid by private supplemental insurance that Medicare beneficiaries carried; approximately 65 percent had such additional coverage. The low average percentage of costs for the elderly under Medicare resulted from the fact that it provided only limited coverage for nursing home care, prescription drugs and eyeglasses. Nursing home care, although it involves a heavy component of medical care, may be primarily a social service rather than a medical service.

The major burden of the Medicare system is created by the very elderly, those who are in the last years of their lives. While approximately 77 percent of the elderly use Medicare at a rate that requires less than $500 per year, 8.8 percent require payments of $3,000 or more a year and consume 70 percent of Medicare's expenditures. All told, the elderly use 31.4 percent of the nation's health care resources, although they constitute only 11.2 percent of the population.[163]

Medicare in 1982 actually paid 75 percent of all the hospital costs of the elderly and 56 percent of physician fees. In 1966, the elderly paid $300 out of pocket for health care costs, above insurance reimbursements, while in 1977 they paid nearly $700, although when these data were adjusted for inflation the difference was small.

The trustees for the Medicare program in 1983 reported, as they had nearly every year since the program's inception, that the fund would run out of money by the end of the 1980s because the tax that financed the hospital part of the program was not keeping pace with the increases in the cost of hospital care. Those increases, which the trustees expected would continue at about 13 percent a year, included not only the general cost of goods in the economy at large, such as wage increases, but also an increase in both the elderly population and the amount of care given to each person admitted to the hospital. This latter, the intensity-of-care item, which was an important factor in the debate over Carter's hospital cost containment legislation, was very tricky to evaluate. It could account for increases in both the quality of care and redundancy of care—excessive tests and the rest. The higher cost of hospital care as a result of newer technology was calculated to be approximately 5 percent of the total. General increases in prices and wages in the economy account for 5.3 percent of the increase in hospital costs, while the increase in the elderly population generally and the number of admissions accounted for 2.5 percent.[164]

There are three generally accepted ways federal health policy-makers can try to correct the problems—they can restrict eligibility to Medicare, they can reduce its benefits, or they can increase its revenues. But there is also a fourth—they can redesign Medicare to focus on outpatient rather than inpatient care.

Medicare revenues are derived from a payroll tax that is lumped together with the social security tax, and a periodic increase in this tax is mandated by law. Eligibility for Medicare is generally linked to eligibility for social security, and as the latter is modified so probably will be the former.

That leaves, of the three generally accepted ways to cut back costs, a cap on benefits, and while the Reagan administration did not, at least by mid-1983, propose modifying benefits per se—that is, it did not support denying treatment already covered—it did propose having the beneficiary pay more. If hospitalized, the beneficiary, under Reagan's 1983 plan, would pay part of the cost of each day in the hospital; for the cost of care by a physician, the beneficiary would pay a higher premium.

One way to increase revenues as yet only lightly considered, briefly by the Finance Committee in 1980 in another context, would be to levy a consumption tax on those who mistreat their health care by what they consume—for example, cigarettes and alcohol. A significant excise tax could be added to those items to help defray Medicare costs. Another method would be to divert part of the gasoline tax to the Medicare trust fund since automobile accidents cause so many injuries. Not only would an increase in alcohol and cigarette taxes provide more revenue for the Medicare trust fund, but it would also cause some people to reduce their consumption of these items, thus perhaps reducing their health care needs. In 1983 the estimated cost of additional health care as a result of alcohol and smoking was $37 billion.

But a fourth, more radical, approach will have to be adopted eventually if the program is to stay afloat. Medicare is now an old-fashioned system based on old-fashioned concepts. It overemphasizes acute-care treatment, and treatment in hospitals, along with the use of high technology to correct the ailment, and it does this while underplaying the desirability of and need for preventive health care and long-term nursing care. The problems Medicare now has to deal with were not present in their current intensity when the program was enacted in 1965. Then acute care was more important. But the intervening years have brought substantial changes in medical care that have made the approach obsolete.

The way most medical care is organized in this country today—primary-care physicians practicing alone or in small groups, associated with one or more hospitals, referring their patients to one or more specialists as the need arises, each entity keeping its own medical records and often with little consultation among the various practitioners treating a particular patient—is, despite its disorganization, in most instances adequate to the needs of the usually healthy and able bodied. But it is not adequate to the needs of the very elderly. The existing system places the responsibility for initiating medical care on the patient, yet the very elderly are often unable to do that. This group needs a system that will, in the words of a 1979 booklet by the National Institute on Aging, "generate appropriate medical attention as well as implement and pay for the needed health . . . services."[165]

Medicare is the wrong system for the elderly, at least the very elderly, who need more than attention here and there for periodic episodes of illness or injury. Instead, a system that has available within a single organization the various medical disciplines that may be called upon to treat the elderly, that contains a unified set of records on the patient, and that has the capacity to reach out to the patient, to see him or her and deliver treatment before the situation becomes critical, is the type of system that should be available, universally, to elderly patients. It is the type of system that has been used by the community health center, the community mental health center and the health maintenance organization. These are prototypes, yet they have largely been ignored by Medicare.

Medicare needs to be redesigned to provide incentives for physicians and other health care practitioners to develop systems of integrated care for the very elderly—systems that pay attention to the broad range of their needs as they move closer to death rather than that simply pay attention to the technological procedures that may provide them with relief for a moment. As the population of the very elderly steadily increases, such a shift in the way Medicare works will become even more imperative.

Health Insurance for the Unemployed

In 1983, even though Ronald Reagan was successful in building more constraints into the Medicare program, he was confronted with a serious effort to create another federally backed health insurance program, this one for unemployed workers. The momentum for this effort was created by the high unemployment rate that had developed during his tenure.

Congress, in fact, by the spring of 1983 had put enactment of a program of health insurance for the unemployed on the fast track, with both Democrats and Republicans agreeing that the problem was serious enough that something should be done to ease the hardship. It was a suggestion with which the White House would reluctantly concur.

But to stay on the fast track, there was a big slippery spot that had to be avoided—ensuring that in the end the new program did not help more than the unemployed without health insurance and that it did not create pressure for a broader, more comprehensive federal health care program. It was a difficult path to tread, and members on both sides of the Capitol, on both sides of the aisle and in each ideological corner were not sure they could do it.

By spring there were more than 11 million people actively seeking work and perhaps another 2 million who wanted work but had given up trying to find a job. It was impossible to determine accurately how many of these workers were without health insurance, for some had been able to retain coverage through their old jobs or from a spouse who was still working, but the Congressional Budget Office estimated that about 10 million people—unemployed workers and members of their families—were then without health insurance because of the recession.

The problem was largely of Ronald Reagan's own making, on two counts. The first was, of course, that his policies had so undermined the economy that the country was experiencing the largest unemployment rate since before World War II. The second was that Reagan's changes in the fabric of federal support for health care had substantially diminished the insulation protecting the federal government from large outcries for expanded involvement in the delivery and financing of health care, such as national health insurance.

All of these schemes affecting the way health care was financed and delivered that had been built up over the years were, as we have seen, the main reason no significant additions had been made to the federal government's support system for health in the past decade and a half. Until unemployment began to swell that number, there was only about 20 million people without some sort of health insurance, and they were for the most part an unorganized constituency. But Reagan's changes, endorsed by Congress, upset that precarious balance.

To respond to the problem of those who were both uninsured and unemployed, Congress decided to add another strand to the existing health care safety net.

Access to health insurance in the United States, as we have seen, is largely derived through employment, and when a person becomes unemployed or is isolated from that arena because a family member is unemployed, he or she loses that access, or at least it becomes more expensive and more difficult. And it is health insurance that guarantees a person access to costly health care services, particularly hospital care.

Surrounding the employment-based health insurance system is a health care safety net, although the strands are different sizes and each one has its own inequities. For the retired, the net consists of Medicare. The disabled who cannot work also have access to Medicare. The poor on welfare, those also not working because jobs are not available to them, have, in many cases, Medicaid. But for the unemployed receiving unemployment compensation, and thus for the most part not qualifying for welfare and thus for Medicaid, there was no strand in the health care safety net—and that was the strand Congress wanted to weave.

There were other strands missing in this safety net as well, primarily ones for the 20 million Americans who did not have health insurance for any number of reasons—they were self-employed, their employers did not provide insurance, they had low incomes but not low enough to qualify for Medicaid. There were others, mostly those who had grossly inadequate health insurance converage. It was this group that congressional health leaders had to bar from entering the health care safety net if they were to write a health insurance program for the unemployed that would be acceptable to most members of Congress and the president. And it was this group, as we have seen, that Congress, whenever it debated health programs, national health insurance or otherwise, always had the most difficulty covering, for they were the most costly to cover.

Over the years as Congress debated the possibility of national health insurance it had come to a tacit understanding that the major burden of any federally mandated expansion of health care services would have to be carried by the employer, thus relieving the federal government of as much expense as possible. That was the tack being pursued again in the summer of 1983 in developing a program of health insurance for the unemployed.

There were initially basically two, largely similar proposals before Congress. The House version was a product of the combined efforts of the Commerce and Ways and Means committees. The other proposal was written by the Senate Finance Committee. The administration, which minimized the seriousness of the situation, had its views, but it did not offer a bill.

Office of Management and Budget Director David Stockman, testifying before the Senate Finance Committee in late April 1983, argued that the number of people threatened with inadequate health insurance because they were unemployed was not nearly as great as the 10 million suggested by CBO. "The problem of lack of health insurance among the unemployed," Stockman said, "is one of selective gaps and discontinuities—and not a pervasive or general problem." The number of long-term unemployed "wholly without access to health care services," he went on, "is really a limited subset of the unemployed." They numbered about 2.1 million, he maintained.[166]

The needs of most uninsured people, he argued, could be met by giving them greater access to employer programs. Once that access was opened up, he said, whatever gaps in coverage remained could be filled by letting states use funds from the social services block grant created in 1981. If Congress did not take this into account when drafting legislation, Stockman went on, it could be a "costly mistake," for pressure would develop to fold into the new program those who did not then have coverage for reasons other than that they are unemployed.

Federal funds under each of the two congressional bills would be made available to states either to purchase health insurance for the unemployed or to pay directly for care they received. Most of the cost would be borne by the federal government. Benefits were similar to those under Medicaid—essential hospital and physician care was covered, but little more. Anyone on the unemployment rolls when the legislation was enacted, or whose unemployment benefits had expired, would be eligible provided he or she did not otherwise have access to health insurance. Participation by a state under either proposal would be voluntary, and each unemployed worker's participation in the program would be voluntary. Also, states could require unemployed workers to pay part of the cost of the insurance as well as part of the cost of care. Both programs would end in a few years. The House proposal did go further—it provided grants to public hospitals—the city- or country-run institutions that get the indigent seeking health care, for their burden has increased as workers loss their insurance. The Senate bill paid for the program by making additional cuts in the Medicare and Medicaid programs. The House bill paid for the program by taking the necessary cash out of the general revenues of the Treasury, an approach that brought a veto threat by the White House.

Both bills required employers to carry health insurance for awhile for former employees and required employers to open up their programs to spouses of employees who lose their jobs.

As the bills were sent to the floor in both the House and Senate by midsummer, the big hurdle facing the lawmakers at the beginning of the year had been overcome. The bills applied only to the unemployed—no one else without health insurance would be eligible. Final action on the measure was put off until the fall. The only thing that seemed to stand in its way was a marked reduction in unemployment; if the rate by fall were to drop significantly Congress might to choose to ignore the legislation in the belief that the problem had been mooted. That was what had happened in 1974 when similar legislation had been considered.

The Senate by choosing to pay for the new program by capturing funds from Medicare and Medicaid had averted another problem that had been identified when it had first taken up the proposal. Originally the Senate had given serious consideration to raising the money for the program by putting a cap on tax deductions by employers for health insurance for their employees. Since not all workers would forgo that broader coverage, some would decide to pay the extra tax imposed. That would raise revenues for the Treasury, and it was these funds that proponents of the Senate bill said initially should be used to pay the additional cost of providing health insurance for the unemployed.

But that approach carried political pitfalls. Many Americans, with broad health insurance coverage for which they paid little or nothing, had come to view well-financed care as an inalienable right. Should they lose even part of that fringe benefit, it could cause trouble; they might want the federal government to take up the slack.

That's what Robert Packwood, a Republican senator from Oregon, was worried about. During the April hearing by the Finance Committee he was very critical of the administration's plan to put a limit on the amount of tax-free health insurance benefits that an employer could provide an employee. If the cap was successful in getting people to scale back their health insurance coverage, he said, workers would "turn and snap at us" for taking away their lucrative fringe benefits and "we will be pushed toward developing a national health insurance program—you will end up with NHI if you go down that road."[167]

In that case, Reagan would have opened up a Pandora's box that he naively thought he had firmly closed.

The Technological Imperative—and Warp

Whether or not a national health insurance program is ever enacted, the federal government, because of its substantial, and rising, investment in health each year will continue to remain the most important force in the nation's health care industry. How the federal investment is made and how the resources are allocated will determine, by and large, the kind and quality of health care almost everyone gets, regardless of who pays the bill. But despite this substantial leverage, federal health policymakers, regardless of the administration in office, have not sought to use it to the fullest extent possible. The focus has instead increasingly been on how to stem the rising tide of inflation, and the cost of health care today remains the major issue. Although this cost, which in the aggregate in 1982 was nearly $325 billion, is characterized by many as too high, the public seems to want more resources spent on medical care and gives a high priority to the growth of investment in this area, higher than in education or other major social programs.

As a consequence, both the federal government and the health care industry are under pressure to pursue bigger and better cures. It is a pressure that gives hospitals and doctors impetus to purchase the best and most recently developed equipment available and to provide the most exotic treatment available, and it is a pressure that renders it difficult for the federal government to make any substantial change in the nature of its commitment in the health care area.

Theodore Cooper, HEW assistant secretary for Health for Presidents Nixon and Ford and himself a physician, has described the dilemma this way:

> We cannot continue to make the citizenry health conscious, disease concerned, symptom aware and expect them not to seek some attention. We cannot continue to tell workers and beneficiaries that they are entitled to more health benefits (in lieu of income), to sell them multiple insurance policies that encourage the use of inpatient resources, and then say we didn't mean for it to cost money. We cannot continue to insist on more dignified personal care with only single or double rooms, with high density nursing, better food service and the "best and newest" of equipment, higher wages for staff and then say we should be able to have these

> improvements at a standard price that is different from that of prices in the rest of the economy. And we cannot continue to enfold new social problems into the medical care system for their attention (like new programs at hospitals for compulsive gamblers) and expect service costs to go down.[168]

How then is it possible to determine whether the investment is too much, too little, or just right?

Indeed, why should the national investment in health care be put to such a test? We do not question the total comparable investment in automobiles or even in transportation, in housing or in candy, cosmetics or food. Is it because health care is considered by some to be a "right" of the individual, and thus should be obtainable by all? Yet housing and food might seem more appropriately such a right.

Rather, the cost of health care and the investment is questioned because of the federal government's large involvement.

Because of the unique nature of health care, it is impossible to determine whether costs today are unreasonable. The health care we buy today is a much different product, by and large, from what we bought several years ago, and in many areas it is much more sophisticated and effective. This new level of treatment costs more. The rise in hospital costs, which is the most dramatic area of health care inflation, over the past decade, therefore, represents in part—in large part, some argue—an increase in the quality as well as the quantity of hospital services.

The drive for ever better health care promotes further technological achievement, but that in turn tends to compound the problem and thwart the final solutions. It is also an area where there are huge amounts of money involved.

Technological advances are a concern because they often only partly solve the problem, or go only halfway, and this halfway technology is a major factor in the rise of health care costs. Lewis Thomas, a physician who is chancellor of the Memorial Sloan-Kettering Cancer Center in New York City, first described the phenomenon in a 1974 essay, "The Technology of Medicine," which today is still the cornerstone of the debate.

Halfway technology, Thomas said, represents the "kinds of things that must be done after the fact, as efforts to compensate for the incapacitating effects of certain diseases whose course one is unable to do very much about. It is a technology designed to make up for disease, or to postpone death."[169]

Halfway technology for chronic kidney failure means expensive dialysis or transplantation; for heart disease the halfway technology is open heart surgery, a pacemaker, a transplant or an artificial heart; for diabetes it is continuing, lifelong treatment. The cost in each of these instances, as well as of others, is substantial. Kidney dialysis costs about $24,000 a year, a coronary bypass about $15,000, implantation of a pacemaker about $10,000. To each of the individuals who benefit from such a procedure the investment is clearly worth the price—and more, much more—regardless of who pays. So it is to family and friends. But for each 90-year-old man who gets a pacemaker paid for by Medicare there are hundreds of poor kids getting little or no health care—and that probably has long-term consequences.

John Cooper, president of the American Association of Medical Colleges, in 1973 congressional testimony described halfway technology as not "really evidence of success in dealing with disease," but rather "confessions of failure, of a lack of understanding to prevent disease before clinical signs and symptoms appear. They are the consequences of a partial understanding."[170]

Polio is perhaps the best example of how a halfway technology was first developed, then resolved. At first polio was a cheap disease, economically. The patient either died or got well without much help and probably was crippled. Then research provided the techniques to sustain the life of those with polio by the use of respirators and other complicated devices. As a consequence, the cost of treating polio rose, and the cost of maintaining those who survived rose, too. Ultimately, however, biomedical research produced a vaccine, and now the disease, by and large, has been eliminated. For all practical purposes, the attendant costs have also been eliminated.

It is only through biomedical research, the foundation of modern health care, that those obstacles can be overcome, that it is possible to move through high technology to a solution. "Through advances in knowledge we can develop the understanding of the living process and its modification by illness required to permit control of disease through prevention of diagnosis and treatment in its earliest, least harmful and least expensive phases," the AAMC's John Cooper said. The important link between medical research and medical costs, he argued, is the ability to "intervene before clinical signs and symptoms appear."[171] Only then would it become possible to control a disease. The most significant value of the federal government in dealing with health care costs, therefore, may be its ability to help the health care industry move through halfway technology to the final phase of full prevention. But at that point, long-term care for the elderly, who are likely to become increasingly feeble as they get older, will become a more critical problem than it is now.

The renal dialysis program is a prime example of how medical technology has saved lives, and how the federal government has absorbed the costs of such care. It is one of two federal programs that covers treatment costs for all who have a specific disease. (The other disease for which the federal government pays the cost of virtually all treatment is Hansen's, or leprosy, but this program works differently. The responsibility for care rests with the Public Health Service, not the Health Care Financing Administration as with renal dialysis, and it pays only for the treatment of Hansen's, not of all other ailments a person may have. Furthermore, the cost of treatment is substantially less.)

Because the renal dialysis program provides nearly universal coverage for treatment of kidney failure it eliminates the private medical market as a basis for setting reimbursement rates. In doing so, it represents, as one report noted, a "unique instance in which the federal government is simultaneously attempting to guarantee near universal access to medical care, control the cost of delivering that care and insuring the delivery of high quality care," all of those things the government would be expected to do if it enacted a comprehensive national health insurance program run and financed by the federal government.[172]

The germ for the program was born in 1967 when the Bureau of the Budget, the predecessor of today's Office of Management and Budget, created a Committee on Chronic Renal Disease that proposed a national program designed to provide treatment, either through dialysis or transplantation, for everyone needing it.

But the program was not authorized by Congress until 1972, and then with very little thought. That was the year Congress enacted legislation making substantial changes in Medicare involving extending benefits to the disabled. Vance Hartke, then a Democratic senator from Indiana, offered an amendment to the social security legislation to have Medicare pay the costs of treating kidney disease. Everyone contributing to the social security program would be covered. Costs were extremely difficult to project, but at the time only about seven thousand persons were getting treatment, and Hartke estimated the initial costs would be about $75 million a year, an estimate that was to prove to be enticingly deceptive.

Neither the House nor the Senate held hearings on the proposal. After Hartke's amendment was adopted by the full Senate, on a Saturday morning in September 1972 following a thirty-minute debate, it went directly to a House-Senate conference committee. There, on a Saturday evening, two weeks later, just before Congress adjourned, the Hartke amendment was put into the final version of the bill.

The only time federal payment of the cost of kidney dialysis had been considered by a congressional committee was in a different context a year earlier when the House Ways and Means Committee was holding hearings on national health insurance. Then, advocates of having NHI cover the cost of dialysis wheeled a patient into the hearing room where he underwent dialysis. It was startlingly effective testimony and has long been remembered by Capitol Hill watchers, but often incorrectly recalled. It did not provide, as many have suggested, the immediate impetus for the legislative authority for the renal dialysis program, but it surely had an effect on those Ways and Means members who a year later were to encounter the provision in conference—they accepted the new program with hardly a murmur.

Nevertheless, kidney disease had been a concern to Wilbur Mills, then the chairman of Ways and Means. For some time he had been badgered by constituents and others to help find treatment for an ailing relative or friend, and thus kidney disease for him came to be associated with names and faces—faces that would lose their color and names that would go on gravestones if help were not provided. In fact, Mills had in previous years sponsored his own legislation to provide for federal payment for treatment of end-stage renal disease, although in a different way than finally adopted. What is more, the original impetus for Russell Long's catastrophic health insurance proposal when it was first proposed in 1970 had been kidney failure; this was a group that desperately needed catastrophic coverage to help pay for cost of treatment.

Instead of the $75-million cost predicted by Hartke, that first year of Medicare coverage for treatment of kidney disease, 1974, the cost was $283 million. In 1980 the cost was $1.4 billion for 64,000 people, and the ultimate patient load, as about 8,000 persons were added to the rolls each year, was expected to level off at nearly 90,000 by 1986, with costs running about $3.1 billion a year.[173]

The annual dialysis cost per patient is approximately $24,000, about $5,000 more than a transplant operation costs. But not all of these costs are exclusively for treatment of kidney disease, for when a kidney patient becomes eligible for Medicare all health care costs are covered just as they are for elderly Medicare patients. Kidney patients constitute less than 0.25 percent of all persons eligible for Medicare, yet they receive more than 10 percent of Medicare part B reimbursements.

Although costs in the program have risen, the rise has been largely due to the increased number of beneficiaries, not to an increase in the costs of treatment. In fact, there has been a remarkable stability in annual beneficiary payments that suggest that the program's costs are not out of control.

Despite its high costs, the renal dialysis program is viewed as successful in more than just a medical sense; it is viewed as one that has found the right combination of economics. Although the cost per patient to Medicare increased between 1974 and 1979, when adjusted for inflation the costs actually have fallen.

The renal dialysis program does have some important features and experience to offer in building a more comprehensive program. Reimbursements to physicians are made through the facilities on a capitation basis, and thus depart from traditional fee-for-service reimbursement. There is de facto mandatory assignment that effectively prevents facilities from billing patients for more than Medicare's allowable deductible and copayment amounts. Also, there is a system of certifying facilities that regulates the number and capacity of treatment and makes sure that their growth is in relation, pretty much, with the patient population.

At first, although both dialysis and transplantation were acceptable treatments, the bias of the program was toward dialysis, and dialysis performed in a hospital, although it could be done both in outpatient treatment centers and, for some, at home. Hospital dialysis was the more costly procedure. In 1978 legislation was enacted providing incentives to treat the problem through transplantation and, if a transplant was not possible, to carry out the dialysis at home, and since then costs per patient have declined slightly.

But there still are worries. The Health Care Financing Administration (HCFA), the federal agency that runs Medicare and thus the end-stage renal dialysis (ESRD) program, in 1980 acknowledged that the "high and steadily rising cost of the program" would cause serious problems for the Medicare trust fund "unless steps are taken to make it more cost-effective."[174]

The program, in fact, is a vivid portrayal of other problems the nation will face in health care treatment if the cost of some procedures like renal dialysis are taken over by the federal government, for it makes a very, very expensive life-saving treatment available to all those who need it, largely at public expense. As aptly described by a 1980 HCFA report, the program encapsulates a familiar dilemma: "Affirming that life is beyond price may carry with it a high social cost. Such ethical considerations lie close to the surface of all policy discussions of this program, never receding, always reminding us of our technical and clinical prowess, our finite resources, our mortality."[175]

The kidney dialysis program has also resulted in the development of a very substantial industry. Equipment and supplies for renal dialysis treatment include the basic machinery, the dialyzers, the dialyzate or fluid that is necessary to operate them, plus ancillary materials such as drugs, needles and syringes, and the monitoring of all this equipment. All told, annual sales for equipment for renal dialysis amount to $300 million a year, all for a population in 1982 of less than 65,000 persons. What is more, the industry is highly concentrated. The three largest dialysis-equipment manufacturing firms have more than 70 percent of the market. One of the biggest firms in the industry, a conglomerate that operates many different medical care ventures, National Medical Care, had gross revenues of $245.5 million in 1982.

It is difficult, therefore, to see the way out of the woods of the Medicare renal dialysis program. The momentum of the present is to give dialysis to all those who need it, and although the program managers believe the ESRD population will taper off at about 90,000, there is no firm way of knowing this. The dialysis population has increased steadily over the years, exceeding early anticipated targets where it was thought it would level off, and as medicine learns more about coping with the non-kidney ailments of ESRD patients, their chance of living longer—and thus the total ESRD population—grows. Now, many dialysis patients are expected to live as long as their contemporaries.

Thus, without a solution to the problem of kidney disease—which is the cause of nearly two-thirds of all kidney failure—there is little chance of working out of the problem, and federal funding for research on kidney disease has remained at a plateau in recent years despite developments that a breakthrough may be on the horizon.

Another possible solution, or at least partial solution, to the dilemma is more transplants. The 1967 Bureau of the Budget committee anticipated that a greater use of transplants would be made than has turned out to be the case. The ideal transplant kidney comes from a living relative, in which case the chance for success is about 90 percent. Most transplants have to come from cadavers, though, in which case the chance for success is only about 55 percent. When a transplant fails—and not every dialysis patient is a good candidate for the operation—the person may have more difficulty on dialysis than before, so there are risks.

Nevertheless, transplants have not been widely used, and in 1980 only about 27 percent of the ESRD population received transplants, slightly fewer than the year before. It is not clear why there is such a lack of popularity with transplants, but cynics point out that every successful transplant removes a patient from dialysis, which means a cut in income of about $24,000 a year for that dialysis facility. It is an awkward suggestion, and perhaps unfair, but there is clearly the chance of considerable reduction in income for dialysis facilities if transplantation were to be more widely used.

The triple coronary bypass is a medical procedure of a different category. It is a highly complicated operation but involves no unusual pieces of medical equipment. And it is one of the most successful operations performed today—the best known of the high-tech procedures. It is a very reliable procedure for lengthening the life of many persons with heart disease, patients with severe blockage of the three arteries that supply the heart muscle or blockage of the left main artery where the three branches originate. The total cost of the operation, which is quite safe, is about $15,000, and for people who need it there is little argument that it is a worthwhile investment. Without the operation they are likely to die; with it they can go on to live productive, active lives.

Some people, however, with less than severe blockage, undergo a modified and less severe operation to gain relief from chest pain caused by an insufficient supply of blood to the heart. This ailment often can be treated as satisfactorily by drugs or other therapy, or by modifying the person's activity; the operation may not be required to save the patient's life, and thus falls into the category of unnecessary use of very expensive health care.

In April 1981, a National Institutes of Health conference on coronary bypass surgery raised a number of important questions about the operation. One speaker, surveying the full gambit of bypass operations, asked why a $2-billion annual investment in a medical procedure that "prolongs life for some and markedly improves life for others" was being questioned when we don't "question the share of our resources going for candy and stereo sets." We do not question the money spent for candy because that is people's own money, he added, while the coronary artery bypass (CAB) funds are in some way subsidized by the federal government. Probably people having to pay the cost out of their own pockets for the CAB would do so, because of the high return.[176]

Much of the federal subsidization of the operation is made through the Medicare program, which pays for bypass surgery for its beneficiaries: those 65 years of age and older, ESRD patients and the disabled. And a disproportionate amount of Medicare CAB payments go to people who are under 65 years of age, primarily the disabled. In 1980, 27 percent of Medicare patients in Maryland getting CABs were under 65, while only 10 percent of all Medicare beneficiaries were under 65. In contrast, only 15 percent of all CABs were performed on people over 65.

But if the coronary bypass is the most successful heart operation, the transplant is the most dramatic and the least successful.

Heart disease kills over one million people in the United States annually, and although transplants have proven somewhat successful, only about fifty such operations are tried each year, largely because of a shortage of organs and the problems of rejection. A heart transplant operation now costs about $125,000.

But heart transplants fell into disfavor because of their high cost and high risks, and probably because of the unique role of the heart in the human, both physical and spiritual; the success rate was very low. In response to this the American College of Surgeons in 1977 discontinued its register of these operations as a way of showing its disfavor. By that time 346 operations had been performed worldwide on 338 patients, with only 77 still living.

The best-known heart transplant team is at Stanford University, and its success is largely due to the fact it has been able to minimize infection. The head of the program, Norman Shumway, performed 281 transplants between 1968 and 1980. Sixty-five percent survived for one year and 40 percent for five; one man lived eleven years.

But the heart transplant, as with other organ transplants, may one day become a thing of the past. Artificial organs that won't be rejected by the human body are being developed, and when perfected may become widely used. An operation in 1969 by Denton Cooley in Houston put the first artificial heart into a human patient, and in 1981 Cooley tried again. Although the patients died, experience showed that it was possible to sustain life temporarily with an artificial heart. Then, on December 2, 1982, Barney Clark successfully was given an artificial heart in a Salt Lake City hospital, and opened up a dramatic new era in heart operations, one that had forebodings of leading the federal government into a different arena similar to the renal dialysis program. Clark lived until March 1983.

Because of the high cost of heart transplants, the federal government from the beginning was induced to pay for all or part of the costs, but it found itself being drawn into a situation where it could end up paying the full costs of all operations, and it sought to prevent this.

By 1979 the Stanford Medical Center was doing half of all transplant operations performed in the United States, or about 25 annually. In November of that year the Department of Health and Human Services authorized Medicare coverage for heart transplants at Stanford in part because it expected to get information upon which to base a final decision regarding Medicare coverage of the operation. But in June 1980, Health and Human Services Secretary Patricia Harris announced that Medicare would no longer pay for heart transplants performed at Stanford until the department had devised an acceptable definition of what constituted a "reasonable and necessary" operation. HHS found "many unresolved issues for which current information is not sufficient," Harris said.[177]

The federal government's decision to withdraw its tentative approval for heart transplants at Stanford was based not on any dissatisfaction with the center's performance, but on the realization that the department had not established sufficiently clear guidelines defining the circumstances under which heart transplant operations would qualify for Medicare coverage.

This decision was also apparently prompted by the ruling of an administrative law judge that directed Medicare to pay for a heart transplant performed at the University of Arizona Medical Center, thus opening up the possibility that Medicare would be required to pay for the operation at any number of hospitals. Harris went on: "There are too many unanswered questions to justify a final decision on general Medicare coverage. These include the patient selection process, the long term social, economic and ethical consequences of the procedure, and the potential for national expansion for the heart transplantation procedure."[178]

In short, the department became worried about its ability to make valid and fair selections as to who should receive the operation and feared the possibility of another federal commitment to a very expensive medical procedure for virtually everyone requesting it, as had happened with the end-stage renal dialysis program. Although it withdrew permission for Stanford to perform heart transplants paid for by Medicare, HHS launched a study of the various issues involved in the procedure.

A Giant Industry

If the United States as a nation today spends, by whatever standard, too much on medical care, this is largely due to the fact that we are spending large hunks of money on procedures like renal dialysis, coronary bypass and heart transplants and on such medical equipment as the CAT scanner.

The problem is not, however, that we spend too much money on medical care, but how we spend it. From an economic point of view, it would clearly be better to spend $3.1 billion a year (which we will soon be spending annually to treat patients with kidney failure) on pregnant women, infants and youths. There, the payoff, in simple economic terms, would be substantial. Yet this is not a decision our political system is capable of making, and understandably so.

To say that we should terminate treatment for renal dialysis patients because, even with treatment, they might live only a few years, is cruel, even murderous. Yet we make the same decision, in a different way, about unborn children and about infants and youths who are presently in good health; we have decided not to provide them with the best possible health care that might help ensure their reasonably good health throughout their lives.

There is much more at stake, though, than the 63,000 people presently undergoing renal dialysis. The industry that has been built up to support that program is huge. And when one looks beyond the treatment of kidney ailment to the rest of the high-tech medical industry, one finds a very large economic undertaking. There is more pressure, in an economic sense, to keep this industry going than to provide periodic checkups for children and youth, and that is a very real part of the problem.

It is extremely difficult to draw an accurate picture of the size of the medical equipment industry; indeed, it is difficult to draw a picture of the size of the health industry generally.

The health industry is often referred to as the nation's third-largest industry, a conclusion based on its share of the gross national product, the number of people employed and a few other bits of similar raw data. The only quantitative figure generally used in government reports is the amount spent for health care in the nation, which in 1981 was $287 billion, or 9.8 percent of the gross national product. By 1982, federal data showed, the investment had grown to $322 billion, or 10.5 percent of the gross national product.[179]

Of the $287 billion spent in 1981 on health care, according to the way the Department of Health and Human Services develops its data, $255 billion went for personal health care provided by hospitals (which took nearly half of this amount), physicians and other health professionals, nursing homes, and for drugs, eyeglasses and other types of health care appliances.

Of the remaining $32 billion, about one third was for administration, $7 billion was for governmental public health activities, $5.7 billion for research and $7.5 billion for construction of health facilities.

In 1980, $12.1 billion was spent for medical devices and diagnostic products—everything from wheelchairs to CAT scanners. That same year health insurance companies, including Blue Cross and Blue Shield, paid out $64 billion in benefits. In 1980, there were more than 1,200 drug manufacturing firms in the country and over 61,000 pharmacies, and that year the sale of drugs alone was $11.1 billion.

The biggest segment of the health services industry, of course, is the hospital sector. In 1979, there were 6,525 short-stay, community hospitals in the country, with a total of more than one million beds. In 1980, there were nearly 4 million full-time hospital workers. The nursing-home industry is also large, and in 1978 there were nearly 19,000 nursing homes with 1.3 million beds.

In contrast, it is possible to get only a much thinner glimpse of the size of the industry that manufactures health care equipment. For example, the world market for medical equipment of diagnostic imagers such as CAT scanners, nuclear magnetic resonators and the like, according to General Electric, which holds 20 percent of this market, is $3.5 billion. And in addition to the hardware that it sells, GE makes a substantial amount each year in servicing that hardware. The company predicts that this world market will rise to $10 billion by 1990.[180]

A substantial portion of the industry providing care is nonprofit, such as hospitals, but another significant portion, like the equipment-manufacturing sector, is owned by investors, which means that those who invest in it intend to make money off their investment.

Traditionally, the for-profit sector has consisted of the drug industry and the manufacturers of medical devices and equipment, everything from tongue depressors to CAT scanners, plus a few hospitals. In recent years, proprietary hospitals have expanded substantially in number and now constitutes nearly 20 percent of all hospitals. In 1979 they grossed about $13 billion. The largest of the firms that own and manage hospitals—Hospital Corporation of America—had net revenues of $2.1 billion in 1982. Then there are the investor-owned nursing homes, which account for nearly 80 percent of all nursing homes, which altogether grossed $15 billion in 1979.

Proprietary-home health care firms grossed nearly $3 billion in 1979, and proprietary laboratory firms grossed about $5 billion.[181]

The health industry is huge and growing. It certainly has an enormous impact on the nation's economy.

All this brings us back to Lewis Thomas's halfway technology discussed earlier. Technology drives health care more and more into the very complicated and very sophisticated hospitals, for they are the only places where the equipment can be supported. And since doctors receive a good part of their training in hospitals, they become used to this equipment and want it available to them when they go out to practice. As Thomas says, "It seems to me an inevitable fact of life that as many of these [combinations of high-tech equipment] as can be will be put together, and as much money as can be found will be spent. I do not see that anyone has much choice in this."[182]

And with investors purchasing stock in General Electric and other equipment makers, the momentum builds to produce more and more equipment. Rarely is the introduction of new medical technology accompanied by an analysis of the benefits. Any improvement is considered good; its cost is rarely considered. Indeed, the equipment itself provides the best insurance that additional equipment will be needed, for many who benefit from this equipment, whose lives are saved, require extra care for the rest of their lives, and their new needs build up pressure for new kinds of equipment. Medicare, which is the single largest spending agent of health care dollars, does not determine whether the funds might be better spent in another way when it approves a new medical procedure for reimbursement.

"The only thing that can move medicine away from this level of technology is new information," says Thomas, "and the only imaginable source of this new information is research."[183]

But in addition to research, the American public will have to come to terms, through our political system, with how we want to use increasingly scarce health resources, and, more important, how aggressively we want to pursue the goal of extending life indefinitely. Although each new development brings us a step closer, in the last analysis it is like trying to square the circle—an impossible task.

EPILOGUE

The two major changes in federal health policy made during the Reagan presidency—the beginning of the dissolution of categorical grant programs and placing firm limits on what the federal government would pay for services to Medicare and Medicaid beneficiaries—were not simply the product of support for Reagan's conservative philosophy but the outgrowth of a number of forces that had begun to generate momentum more than ten years earlier.

Dissatisfaction with categorical grants had surfaced as far back as the latter part of the 1960s. Only a few years after the device had become part of the general scheme of things, Representative Paul Rogers, then a leader in the House on health matters, suggested that targeting federal funds at specific health problems was no longer the best way to proceed; a broader sweep of authority was needed. That call went unheeded, and the process of creating new and specialized grant programs continued through the 1970s, although at a diminishing rate. Early in the Nixon administration both the White House and Congress became increasingly concerned about the rising costs of the Medicare and Medicaid programs, and both in their own way sought to check that rise. They were not successful.

It is possible that both issues would have been dealt with squarely and another health policy system devised had a Democratic president been elected in 1968, but that is unlikely—and of course it did not happen. Republican Nixon was elected, and he had to deal with a Democratic Congress. Ultimately Nixon and Congress worked themselves into a standoff over policy differences, of which health policy was only one. The larger issues were Vietnam, impoundments and Watergate, but they all boiled down to a strong disagreement between a Democratic Congress, somewhat liberal, and a Republican president, somewhat conservative. Even within that context, particularly after Nixon had quit and Gerald Ford was president, signs emerged that congressional Democrats were becoming sympathetic to proposals to soften the federal government's role in the involvement of health care delivery.

As Jimmy Carter became president, the focus of federal health policymakers was increasingly on the problem of rising health care costs, but parallel to that concern was a continued growth of the feeling that categorical grants had outgrown their usefulness. The momentum that had developed meant that change was more or less inevitable, if not during Carter's administration then later.

By the middle of the Carter presidency, the economic buoyancy of the United States was clearly over; the country had shifted into a new era in which it was not able to spend all the money it might want to spend without running into serious budget—and thus, in part, inflation—difficulties. Furthermore, the country generally was becoming more conservative politically, and this was reflected in the makeup of Congress; the House was clearly losing whatever liberal tinge it had, and the Senate would lose its liberal bias in the election of 1980.

The differences between Democratic President Carter and the Democratically controlled Congress during the latter half of the 1970s were not so much in political ideology, as had been the case during the early seventies, and they certainly were not the traditional standoff between a president of one party and a Congress of another. Instead, they flowed from two sources. The first was the institutionalization of Congress that had occurred during the Nixon years, when Congress developed resources that were to be exclusively its own for designing public policy and that culminated, in a sense, with the enactment of the Congressional Budget Act in the summer of 1974. Congress from then on was to exercise institutional independence, and if it went along with the president, as it later would do with Ronald Reagan during his first two years, it would be because the president had the votes.

The second reason for Carter's difficulties was his inability to provide effective leadership. Although Congress had developed this institutional independence, it gave an indication of wanting strong leadership from the White House when it was once again occupied by a Democrat. That did not turn out to be what happened, and Congress showed some disappointment, even frustration and anger. Carter's effort to win enactment of hospital cost containment was a long, tortuous experience that seriously eroded the possibility for a successful working relationship between congressional health leaders and the administration on the development of health policy. Carter, and Califano as HEW secretary in his behalf, tended to stonewall Congress. The belligerency between the two institutions that had been so manifest during the Nixon years now reappeared in another way. Carter's problems were largely of his own making.

It is risky to suggest that one event forced Kennedy to contest Carter for the Democratic nomination in 1980, but clearly the president's handling of national health insurance was a compelling factor in persuading the senator to run. Over and over as I interviewed for this book I heard the same conclusion from people allied with Kennedy, with Carter and in between—Kennedy would not have run had he been able to work out a compromise with Carter on national health insurance. Had that happened, Reagan might not have become president, for the divisiveness of 1980 within the Democratic Party shared heavily in the responsibility for Carter's loss to Reagan.

To the extent that there was an increasingly conservative mood in the country, it helped Reagan and, perhaps even more important, helped turn the Senate over to the Republicans, but it was not, I believe, the decisive factor.

All this having happened, the stage was set for some radical changes in federal health policy, as well as in other areas of public policy, as Reagan came into office, and the new president took advantage of the opportunity. But he was not able to go as far as he would have liked. On health issues, Reagan adopted Ford's policy of dismantling the categorical health grant programs by consolidating them into block grants that would give the states considerable freedom to run the programs as they wished. (Reagan and others described this as returning authority to the states, but it was not a return, for the states had never assumed it; categorical grant programs had been constructed at the federal level precisely because states had failed to exercise responsibility—there were huge needs not being satisifed and the federal government had stepped in to fill the voids.)

And it was time for this to happen. State governments, for a number of reasons—a principal one being the financial support the categorical and other federal programs had provided—had improved substantially their capacity to provide services to their constituents. The categorical grant programs had become too many; they were tripping over each other; they had fostered large bureaucracies that were, at least to some degree, more concerned about preserving their own domain than they were about making sure services were successfully delivered to the people who needed them, which was the whole point of these efforts. It was time, in the natural evolution of our political system, to make the change, and that change would have been made regardless of who was president and what the political makeup of Congress had been.

Although rearguard actions were fought against the dismantling of the categorical health grant programs, they were for the most part taken apart. This was a significant change in existing policy, but one, as noted, that was the culmination of an evolutionary process. It would be hard to restore these programs to their previous place of eminence once the political climate changed, but efforts probably will be made to do just that.

Paring back of federal spending for health through Medicare and Medicaid was different in character and would be easier to change as the political leadership changed again. Here the changes, also part of an evolutionary process, were for the most part less radical, although the dollars involved would be greater than with the categorical programs. Caps were imposed on federal spending through these programs by placing limits on what the Medicare program would pay hospitals and physicians. Hospitals, instead of being reimbursed for their cost of providing care to an elderly person, would be told how much they would receive for providing a specific service—replacing a hip, a coronary bypass or removal of a cataract. This was called prospective reimbursement. It was an important change because it placed absolute limits on payments to hospitals and forced them either to find a way to provide the service for what the government would pay or to absorb the difference (and probably find another way to make it up, like charging a higher rate to non-Medicare patients). It was not the Carter hospital cost-containment proposal but it was a step in that direction. In fact, it was similar in many respects to the proposal offered initially during the Ford years by Senator Talmadge to cap Medicare and Medicaid costs, a proposal that Carter spurned.

At the same time, Reagan proposed several other changes in the Medicare program, changes that Congress might take up later. These included placing a limit on the amount that an employer could contribute to a worker's health insurance policy without some of the contribution becoming taxable income to the employee, offering Medicare beneficiaries vouchers with which they could purchase private health insurance policies in lieu of using Medicare, and requiring Medicare patients to pay part of the cost of their hospital care each day they were in the hospital. These proposals were part of a much-touted competition health care plan that Reagan had talked about during the 1980 campaign.

The change in 1983 to a prospective reimbursement system for Medicare was one that everyone—Democrats and Republicans alike—was willing to make. There was no question by early 1983, when the idea was proposed and Congress began working on it, that such a change would have to be made if any degree of integrity for the Medicare program was to be retained, and if the trust fund that financed the program was to be kept from going broke, although that change in and of itself would not stave off bankruptcy. Even more radical surgery would be required.

But the question remained: What would be the next step?

The vacuum in federal involvement in health care left by the Reagan presidency was not likely to result in creation of a dramatic new policy. Instead, the chance was that, as the political complexion of both the White House and Congress changed, old programs would be rebuilt. During the Reagan years, some of the most liberal members of Congress saw themselves as fighting a rearguard action in the health area. Indeed, this is the line that Henry Waxman, chairman of the House Commerce health subcommittee, took when interviewed early in 1983. He said he was not looking into the future and anticipating and preparing for changes that might be made when a Democratic government came to power. Instead, he was concentrating on preserving the old order as much as possible. When the opportunity did arise to make changes he would want to make them slowly.

In 1983, as cracks opened up on the formidable Reagan offensive, retreats to the old order were made. An emergency jobs bill enacted by Congress in the spring of 1983 carried nearly a half-billion dollars to restore funds previously cut out of categorical health programs; they were restored as part of an effort to buttress services to the poor and the unemployed. Other pieces of the old system, such as beefing up the maternal and child health programs, were strengthened. Legislation to enact a program of health insurance for the unemployed was another effort to shore up the existing system. A dramatic shift to a new way of doing things would likely not be made.

It is difficult to make significant changes in federal health policy within the existing governmental and political framework that has in a larger context created barriers to change. With regard to health care the two most distorting forces that warp the system and result in skewed services are insurance and federal tax deductions—insurance because it insulates the patient so heavily from the cost of the services he is receiving to the extent that he may not care what they cost, and the tax system because when health services do cost something the cost may be softened by tax deductions.

A presidential commission in 1983 tackled the question of the federal government's responsibility regarding health care. "Society has an ethical obligation to ensure equitable access to health care for all," concluded the President's Commission for the Study of Ethical Problems in Medicine and Biomedical and Behavioral Research. The obligation, it said, drawing a distinction regarding other human needs, "rests in the special importance of health care; its role in relieving suffering, preventing premature death, restoring functioning, increasing opportunity."[184]

How then to accomplish this?

Any of the major national health insurance programs proposed since the early 1970s—the original Kennedy bill or the one Kennedy proposed in 1974 with Wilbur Mills or the other one he put forward in 1979 with Henry Waxman; Nixon's 1974 plan; or Carter's 1979 plan (particularly the long-term version)—could have accomplished the goals set by the president's commission. But considering the way our political system works, such a sweeping change probably won't be made.

Instead, what is likely is that there will be more efforts—like that of 1983 to provide health insurance for the unemployed—to fill the gaps, to weave more strands into the health care safety net. Slowly, the health care safety net will be strengthened—the unemployed will be covered, a national catastrophic insurance will be instituted, Medicaid will be nationalized and strengthened, employers will be required to provide insurance with minimum standards and to pay a certain amount of the cost, and others not otherwise covered will be brought into the system. As more people are covered, the mandated benefits will be broadened. All this will fill the gaps.

At the same time, the problem of health care costs will probably be tackled differently. To the extent that more competition in the health care marketplace is successful in checking rising costs, Congress and the administration will be deflected from regulatory programs, such as Carter's hospital cost-containment proposal. The core of the marketplace strategy is to put as much of the cost of health care as possible on the employer and the individual, for they are likely to act more quickly than the federal government to say no to higher costs, even if it means foregoing some health care. At the same time, of course, this will save federal dollars—a primary concern of any president or any Congress for decades to come. If competition in the marketplace is not able to do the job by itself, various degrees of federal and/or state regulation are likely.

Whatever steps are adopted, they seem to lead slowly to a reasonably comprehensive and universal national health care system with costs that are somewhat in check. Federal health policy is all about seeing that people who live in this country have access to adequate health care. It is a goal that is often lost in the complexity of the way we carry out our business of government, but it is not a goal that will necessarily get permanently buried.

ABBREVIATIONS

AMA—American Medical Association
CAB—Coronary Artery Bypass
CAT scanner—Computerized axial tomography scanner
CBO—Congressional Budget Office
CHAP—Child Health Assurance Program
CMHC—Community Mental Health Center
CON—Certificate of Need
COWAPS—Council on Wage and Price Stability
CPI—Consumer Price Index
DHEW—Department of Health, Education and Welfare
DHHS—Department of Health and Human Services
EPSDT—Early Periodic Screening, Detection and Treatment
ESRD—End-State Renal Disease
FDA—Food and Drug Administration
HEW—Department of Health Education and Welfare
HHS—Department of Health and Human Services
HMO—Health Maintenance Organization
NHI—National Health Insurance
NIH—National Institutes of Health
NIMH—National Institute of Mental Health
PSRO—Professional Standard Review Organization
SNMA—Student National Medical Association
UAW—United Auto Workers

ACKNOWLEDGMENTS

I am indebted to many people in connection with this book, and those debts go back many years. Harry Schnibbe was the first to expose me to the labyrinths of federal health policy, and his tutelage in the late 1960s served as the foundation upon which my work and reporting were built. Mike Gorman also served as an early teacher and helped me enormously to better understand what was happening, which wasn't always what it seemed to be at first glance. I am indebted to those—more than fifty in number—who generously gave of their time in interviews to describe their experiences in the making of federal health policy as officials in the Executive Branch, members of Congress, congressional staffers, and outside observers and participants. Without their views and insights this book would be much less than it is. I am also indebted to those who read an early version of the manuscript—Mike and Ruth Newman, Chris Koyanagi, Bill Goldman, and Helen Smits—for their exceedingly helpful comments, and to Glenn Markus and Peter Fox who read a later version, both of whom provided many important and constructive suggestions. And I am very, very indebted to my wife, Judy, not only for her reading of the manuscript, both as a layperson to the subject and as a professional writer herself, but also for her support over the three and a half years it took me to write the book. My children, Hugh and Willa, were also very supportive, and tolerant. Nowhere, however, is my debt greater than to Ms. Pross (formally known as TRS 80-II), who repeatedly and without complaint typed the manuscript. Never once did she fail to be available to work when needed. Never once did she blip or blow a circuit and thus lose all the work we had done. And not once did she complain about my inability to proofread and spell accurately—never did she tear her hair or kick the table as my erstwhile editors had done; she simply gracefully pointed out the mistakes and waited for me to correct them. Whatever mistakes, of any kind, remain, of course, are entirely my responsibility.

NOTES

1. *Inaugural Address of the Presidents of the United States* (Washington, D.C.: Government Printing Office, 1974), p. 201.

2. Daniel S. Hirshfield, *The Lost Reform: The Campaign for Compulsory Health Insurance in the United States from 1932 to 1943* (Cambridge, Mass.: Harvard University Press, 1970), chap. 1.

3. *The Public Papers and Addresses of Franklin Delano Roosevelt, 1935* (New York: Random House, 1938), Vol. 4, p. 45.

4. Robert A. Taft, *Congressional Record,* May 3, 1946, p. 4390.

5. *Building America's Health: A Report to the President by the President's Commission on the Health Needs of the Nation* (Washington, D.C., Dec. 18, 1952).

6. Interview with Paul Rogers, Jan. 26, 1983.

7. *Budget of the U.S. Government, FY 1984,* p. 5-103, p. 5-130; *Appendix,* p. IV-103; *Special Analysis,* p. G-627; and Department of Defense press office.

8. *Investigation of HEW,* Report of the Special Subcommittee on Investigation of the Department of Health, Education and Welfare of the Committee on Interstate and Foreign Commerce, U.S. House of Representatives (H Rept 2266), Oct. 13, 1966, p. 16.

9. Ibid., pp. 22f.

10. Ibid., p. 46, p. 49.

11. *Federal Role in Health,* Committee on Government Operations, U.S. Senate (S Rept 91-809), April 30, 1970, p. 29.

12. Ibid., p. 30.

13. Ibid., pp. 30-1.

14. Henry A. Foley, *Community Mental Health Legislation: The Formative Process* (Lexington, Mass.: Lexington Books, 1975), p. 1.

15. *Health Professions Educational Assistance Act of 1963,* Report of the Committee on Interstate and Foreign Commerce, U.S. House of Representatives (HR 12, H Rept. 109), March 19, 1963, p. 9.

16. *Health Professions Educational Assistance Act of 1963,* Report of the Committee on Labor and Public Welfare, U.S. Senate (HR 12, S Rept. 485), Sep. 10, 1963, p. 3.

17. *Department of Health and Human Services FY 1984 Budget,* Details released Jan. 31, 1983, pp. 33, 36.

18. *Congressional Record,* April 7, 1965, p. H7223.

19. Interview with Wilbur Mills, Jan 18, 1983.

20. *CQ Almanac, 1965* (Washington, D.C.: Congressional Quarterly, Inc.), p. 252.

21. *Social Security Amendments of 1965,* Committee on Ways and Means, U.S. House of Representatives (HR 6675, H Rept. 213), March 29, 1965, p. 243.

22. Ibid., p. 253.

23. Data supplied by the Health Insurance Association of America, Washington, D.C.

24. *Medicare and Medicaid: Problems, Issues and Alternatives,* Report of the Staff to the Committee on Finance, U.S. Senate, committee print, Feb. 9, 1970, pp. 1f.

25. *Medicare After 15 Years: Has It Become a Broken Promise to the Elderly?,* Select Committee on Aging, U.S. House of Representatives, committee print, Nov. 17, 1980, p. 2.

26. *Medicare/Medicaid Data Book, 1981,* Health Care Financing Administration, Department of Health and Human Services, April 1982, p. 16, table 2.2, p. 20, table 2.6, and *Department of Health and Human Services, FY 1984 Budget,* p. 33.

27. *Medicare/Medicaid Data Book,* p. 17, table 2.3, and *DHHS FY 1984 Budget,* p. 27, and *End-Stage Renal Disease Program Under Medicare,* Finance Committee Print (CP 97-9), Sept. 1981, p. 40.

28. Finance Committee Print (CP 97-9), p. 40, and *FY 1984 Budget Appendix,* p. I-K 31f.

29. James L. Sundquist, *The Decline and Resurgence of Congress* (Washington, D.C.: Brookings Institution, 1981), pp. 204f.

30. *Public Law 96-296,* sec. 601; June 30, 1970.

31. "Conference Report," *Congressional Record,* June 6, 1970, p. 18960.

32. Richard M. Nixon, "Veto Message," *Weekly Compilation of Presidential Documents* (Washington, D.C.: Office of the Federal Register), June 22, 1970.

33. *NCCMHC et al vs. Caspar Weinberger et al,* Decision by Judge Gerhard A. Gesell, U.S. District Court for the District of Columbia, Aug. 3, 1973; civil action no. 1223-73.

34. Richard M. Nixon, "Message to Congress," *Weekly Compilation of Presidential Documents* (Washington, D.C.: Office of the Federal Register), Feb. 18, 1971.

35. Interview with Max Fine, Sept. 21, 1982.

36. Interview with Larry Horowitz, Jan. 12, 1983.

37. Edward M. Kennedy, remarks on introducing the Health Security Act, *Congressional Record,* Jan. 25, 1971, p. 284.

38. Ibid.

39. Ibid., p. 285.

40. *Health Care Financing Review,* Health Care Financing Administration, Department of Health and Human Services, Sept. 1982 (pub. no. 03146), pp. 19-20, table 1.

41. Richard M. Nixon, "Message to Congress," Feb. 18, 1971.

42. Edward M. Kennedy, Testimony during hearings on National Health Insurance, Committee on Finance, U.S. Senate, April 26, 1971, pp. 32, 545.

43. Ibid.

44. *Journal of the American Medical Association,* Dec. 3, 1932, p. 1951, as quoted in *The Health Maintenance Organization and its Effects on Competition,* Staff Report of the Federal Trade Commission, Bureau of Economics, July 1977, p. 7.

45. Richard M. Nixon, "Press Conference," *Weekly Compilation of Presidential Documents* (Washington, D.C.: Office of the Federal Register), July 14, 1969.

46. Richard M. Nixon, "Message to Congress," *Weekly Compilation of Presidential Documents* (Washington, D.C.: Office of the Federal Register), Feb. 18, 1971.

47. *Towards a Comprehensive Health Policy for the 1970s: A White Paper,* Department of Health, Education and Welfare, May 1971, p. 37.

48. *Health Maintenance Organizations: Comparison of Major Health Maintenance Organization Legislative Proposals,* Committee on Interstate and Foreign Com-

merce, U.S. House of Representatives (committee print no. 14), Feb. 10, 1972, p. 111.

49. *Social Security and Welfare Reform: Summary of the Principal Provisions of HR 1,* Committee on Finance (committee print), June 13, 1972, pp. 23-24.

50. Ibid.

51. *Health Maintenance Organization and Resource Development Act of 1972,* Report of the Committee on Labor and Public Welfare, U.S. Senate (S 3327, S Rept. 92-978), July 21, 1972, p. 2.

52. Ibid.

53. Ibid., p. 1.

54. *Health Maintenance Organization and Resources Act of 1973,* Report of the Committee on Labor and Public Welfare, U.S. Senate (S 14, S Rept. 93-129), April 27, 1973, p. 7.

55. Ibid.

56. Ibid.

57. *Health Maintenance Amendments of 1975,* Committee on Interstate and Foreign Commerce, U.S. House of Representatives (HR 9019, H Rept. 94-518), Sept. 26, 1975, p. 9.

58. Hale Champion, Testimony on *Health Maintenance Organization Act Amendments of 1978 (S 2534),* Hearings before the Subcommittee on Health and Scientific Research of the Committee on Human Resources, U.S. Senate, March 3, 1978, p. 66.

59. *National HMO Development Strategy through 1988,* Public Health Service, Department of Health, Education and Welfare (pub. no. PHS 79-50111), Sept., 1979, accompanying press release dated Oct. 5, 1979, p. 2.

60. *Physicians for a Growing America,* Report of the Surgeon General's Consultant Group on Medical Education [Bane Committee] (Washington, D.C.: Government Printing Office, 1959), p. 12.

61. *Third Report to the President and Congress on the Status of Health Professions Personnel in the United States,* Public Health Service, Department of Health, Education and Welfare, Jan. 1982 (HEW pub. no. HRA 82-2), p. A10, and *Interim Report of the Graduate Medical Education National Advisory Committee,* to the Secretary of the Department of Health, Education and Welfare, April 1979 (HEW pub. no. HRA 79-633), p. 144, table 10.

62. Edward M. Kennedy and Wilbur D. Mills, Joint Statement on Introducing the *Comprehensive National Health Insurance Act of 1974,* April 2, 1974.

63. Interview with Stanley Jones, August 18, 1982.

64. Gerald R. Ford, "Address to a Joint Session of Congress," *Weekly Compilation of Presidential Documents* (Washington, D.C.: Office of the Federal Register), Aug. 2, 1974.

65. *A National Health Insurance Proposal,* Committee on Ways and Means, U.S. House of Representatives (committee print), Aug. 19, 1974.

66. Gerald R. Ford, "Address to the Nation," *Weekly Compilation of Presidential Documents* (Washington, D.C.: Office of the Federal Register), Jan. 13, 1975.

67. *Health, United States, 1982,* Department of Health and Human Services (pub. no. PHS 83-1232), Dec. 1982, p. 134, table 67, p. 136, table 69, and *Statistical Abstract of the United States, 1982–83,* Department of Commerce, Bureau of Census, December 1982, p. 461, table 758, and *Health Care Financing*

Review, Health Care Financing Administration, Department of Health and Human Services (DHHS pub. no. 30146), Sept. 1982, p. 19, table 1, p. 32, table 8, and data collected by the author from the Bureau of Labor Statistics, Department of Labor.

68. *The Complex Puzzle of Rising Health Care Costs: Can the Private Sector Fit it Together,* Council on Wage and Price Stability, Executive Office of the President, Dec. 1976, p. i.

69. Zachary Y. Dyckman, *Physicians: A Study of Physicians' Fees,* Council on Wage and Price Stability, Executive Office of the President, March 1978, p. iii.

70. Ibid., p. vi.

71. Martin S. Feldstein, Testimony on the *Hospital Cost Containment Act of 1979 (S 570),* During hearings before the Committee on Labor and Human Resources, Subcommittee on Health, U.S. Senate, March 15, 1979, p. 290.

72. Jimmy Carter, Speech before the Student National Medical Association, April 16, 1976, as quoted in *Health Systems Report Special Issue on National Insurance and the First Six Months of Carter's Health Policy* [hereafter *HSR Special Issue*] (Washington, D.C.: Morris Inc.), July 1977.

73. Interview with Stephen Schlossberg, December 21, 1982.

74. Jimmy Carter, Statement before the Platform Committee of the Democratic National Committee, June 12, 1976, as reported in *HSR Special Issue,* p. iv.

75. *Health Systems Report* [hereafter *HSR*] (Washington, D.C.: Morris Inc.), July 5, 1976, p. 2.

76. "Health Security Action Committee memorandum," June 16, 1976, as reported in *HSR,* July 5, 1976, p. 2.

77. Interview with Peter Bourne, June 22, 1976, as reported in *HSR,* July 5, 1976, pp. 2f.

78. Jimmy Carter, "Student National Medical Association speech," as reported *HSR Special Issue,* pp. iii, v.

79. Ibid., p. ii.

80. Jimmy Carter, "Presentation before Platform Committee of the Democratic National Committee," as reported *HSR Special Issue,* p. vi.

81. Ibid., p. iii.

82. *Playboy Magazine,* Nov. 1975, as reported in *HSR Special Issue,* p. xiii.

83. Joseph A. Califano, Jr., *Governing America: An Insider's Report from the White House and the Cabinet* (New York: Simon and Schuster, 1981), p. 39.

84. Interview with Stuart Eizenstat, Jan. 4, 1983.

85. Califano, *Governing America,* p. 149.

86. Rogers interview (see note 6).

87. *Congressional Record,* Oct. 12, 1978, pp. S18362, S18391.

88. *HSR,* Oct. 20, 1978, p. 3.

89. Ibid., p. 4.

90. *HSR Almanac 1978,* p. 36.

91. Ibid., p. 9.

92. *National Health Planning and Resources Development Act of 1974,* Report of the Committee on Interstate and Foreign Commerce, U.S. House of Representatives (HR 16204, H. Rept. 93-1382), Sept. 26, 1974, p. 5.

93. *National Health Planning and Development Act of 1974 (S 2994),* Hearings

before the Subcommittee on Health, Committee on Labor and Public Welfare, U.S. Senate, March 11, 1974, Part I, p. 2.

94. Press material, Security Analysts Briefing, General Electric Medical Systems, May 5, 1982, Milwaukee, Wis.

95. Eizenstat interview (see note 84) and Bourne interview, Sept. 15, 1982.

96. Horowitz interview (see note 36).

97. Califano, *Governing America,* p. 100.

98. Ibid., p. 92.

99. Horowitz interview (see note 36).

100. Califano, *Governing America,* p. 106.

101. Ibid., p. 108.

102. Interview with Charles Schultze, Jan. 10, 1983.

103. Califano, *Governing America,* p. 103.

104. Ibid., p. 111.

105. Ibid., p. 113.

106. Fine interview (see note 35).

107. Califano, *Governing America,* pp. 114–16.

108. Author's notes, Aug. 4, 1978.

109. Edward M. Kennedy, Statement on National Health Insurance, July 28, 1978, press release in conjunction with press conference.

110. Stuart Eizenstat, Transcript of July 29, 1978, press conference with Califano on release of national health insurance principles, p. 3.

111. Ibid., p. 2.

112. Edward M. Kennedy, Statement on the floor of the Senate on making public the outline of his new national health insurance program, *Congressional Record,* Oct. 2, 1978, p. S33008.

113. Joseph A. Califano, Jr., Statement before the Committee on Human Resources, U.S. Senate, Oct. 13, 1978, p. 18.

114. Jimmy Carter, "State of the Union Message," *Weekly Compilation of Presidential Documents* (Washington, D.C.: Office of the Federal Register), Jan. 23, 1979.

115. Jimmy Carter, "Message to Congress on Hospital Cost Containment," *Weekly Compilation of Presidential Documents* (Washington, D.C.: Office of the Federal Register), March 6, 1979.

116. Herman E. Talmadge, Statement as reported in *HSR,* March 16, 1979, p. 1.

117. *The Hospital Cost Containment Act of 1979: A Preliminary Analysis* (Washington, D.C.: Congressional Budget Office, May 1979), p. iv.

118. David Stockman, *Congressional Record,* Nov. 15, 1979, p. H10860.

119. Common Cause press release, Dec. 18, 1979.

120. Jimmy Carter, *Keeping Faith: Memoirs of a President* (New York: Bantam Books, 1982), p. 87.

121. Califano, *Governing America,* p. 144.

122. Carter, *Keeping Faith,* p. 87.

123. *Healthy People: The Surgeon General's Report on Health Promotion and Disease Prevention,* Department of Health, Education and Welfare (pub. no. PHS 79-55071), July 1979, p. 1–1.

124. Julius B. Richmond, MD, Statement on Childhood Immunization, Sept. 28, 1979.

125. *Healthy People,* pp. 1–7.

126. C. Everett Koop, MD, Statement in conjunction with release of the 1982 report, *The Health Consequences of Smoking,* of the Department of Health and Human Services, p. 1.

127. *Healthy People,* Secretary's Foreword (addendum, July 26, 1979), p. i.

128. Ibid., p. ii.

129. Russell Long, Statement on the floor of the Senate on introducing his Catastrophic Health Insurance proposal, *Congressional Record,* Feb. 6, 1979, p. S1132.

130. Califano, *Governing America,* p. 129.

131. Ibid., p. 130–31.

132. Edward M. Kennedy, "Health Care Services for all Americans Act," *Congressional Record,* Sept. 6, 1979, p. S12083.

133. *Papers on the Administration of Jimmy Carter, 1979* (Washington, D.C.: Government Printing Office, June 12, 1979), p. 1027.

134. Carter papers, p. 1026.

135. Jimmy Carter, "Message to Congress on his National Health Plan," *Weekly Compilation of Presidential Documents* (Washington D.C.: Office of the Federal Register), June 12, 1979.

136. Joseph A. Califano, Jr., Statement before the Committee on Finance, U.S. Senate, March 27, 1979, p. 2.

137. *HSR,* March 30, 1979, p. 1.

138. Russell Long, *Congressional Record,* June 14, 1979, p. S7680.

139. *Presentation of Major National Health Insurance Proposals,* Hearings before the Committee on Finance, U.S. Senate, June 19, 21, 1979; p. 2.

140. Ibid., p. 3.

141. Ibid., p. 4.

142. Ibid.

143. Ibid., p. 520.

144. Ibid., p. 521, and author's notes.

145. Author's notes.

146. Franklin D. Chu and Sharland Trotter, *The Madness Establishment: Ralph Nader's Study Group Report on the National Institute of Mental Health* (New York: Grossman Publishers, 1974), p. 202.

147. Henry Santiestevan, *Out of Their Beds and Into the Streets* (Washington, D.C.: American Federal of State, County and Municipal Employees, Feb. 1979).

148. Jimmy Carter, Remarks on signing Executive Order 11973, *Weekly Compilation of Presidential Documents* (Washington, D.C.: Office of the Federal Register), Feb. 17, 1977.

149. *Report of the President's Commission on Mental Health,* Washington, D.C.: Government Printing Office, 1978), vol. 1, pp. 17, 4.

150. Ibid., pp. 17f.

151. *Tax Expenditures: Budget Control Options for and Five Year Budget Projections, Fiscal Year 1983–87* (Washington, D.C.: Congressional Budget Office, Nov. 1982), p. 51f, table A-1 (function 551).

152. Ibid.

153. *Tax Subsidies for Medical Care: Current Policies and Possible Alternatives,* Background Paper (Washington, D.C.: Congressional Budget Office, Jan. 1980), p. 25.

154. Alice M. Rivlin, *Tax Expenditures for Health Care,* Hearings before the Task Force on Tax Expenditures and Tax Policy of the Committee on the Budget and the Subcommittee on Oversight of the Committee on Ways and Means, U.S. House of Representatives, July 9, 1979, p. 2.

155. Karen Davis, *Proposals to Restructure the Financing of Private Health Insurance,* Hearings before the Subcommittee on Health, Committee on Ways and Means, U.S. House of Representatives, Feb. 25, 1980, p. 15.

156. Karen Davis, *Proposals to Stimulate Health Care Competition (S 1968),* Hearings before the Subcommittee on Health, Committee on Finance, U.S. Senate; March 18-19, 1980, p. 37.

157. Alice M. Rivlin, Testimony on S1968, p. 29.

158. *HSR,* June 20, 1980, p. 1.

159. John L. Palmer and Isabell V. Sawhill, *The Reagan Experiment* (Washington, D.C.: Urban Institute Press, 1982), p. 294, table 9.5.

160. Carolyne K. Davis, Testimony before the Committee on the Budget, Task Force on Entitlements, Uncontrollables and Indexing, U.S. House of Representatives, March 10, 1983.

161. Palmer and Sawhill, p. 288.

162. Anne R. Sommers, "Rethinking Medicare to Meet Future Needs," paper presented to the Government Research Corporation's 7th Annual Leadership Conference on Health Policy, Washington, D.C., June 17, 1982, p.1.

163. John K. Iglehart, *Rethinking Medicare to Meet Future Needs,* Issues Book [hereafter GRC Issues Book] (Washington, D.C.: Government Research Corporation, 1982), p. 7, box.

164. Wendell E. Primus, GRC Issues Book, p. 9.

165. *Observations on Geriatric Medicine,* National Institute on Aging, Department of Health, Education and Welfare (pub. # NIH-79-162).

166. David Stockman, testimony before the Committee on Finance, U.S. Senate, April 27, 1983.

167. Author's notes.

168. *Competition in the Health Care Sector: Past, Present, and Future* (Washington, D.C.: Federal Trade Commission, March 1978), p. 16.

169. Lewis Thomas, *The Lives of a Cell: Notes of a Biology Watcher* (New York: Bantam Books, 1974), p. 37.

170. John A. D. Cooper, *Medical Policies and Costs,* Hearings before the Subcommittee on Consumer Economics, Joint Economic Committee, U.S. Congress, May 15, 1973, p. 10.

171. Ibid.

172. Richard A. Rettig, *Implementing the End-Stage Renal Disease Program of Medicare* (Santa Monica, Calif,: Rand Corporation, Study prepared for the Health Care Financing Administration, Department of Health, Education and Welfare [R-2505-HCFA/HEW], Sept. 1980), p. 5.

173. *End-Stage Renal Disease (ESRD) Program Under Medicare,* Committee on Finance, U.S. Senate (committee print CP 97-9), Sept. 1981, p. 3.

174. *Medicare Program: Incentive Reimbursement for Outpatient Dialysis and Self-*

Care Dialysis Training (Washington, D.C.: Federal Register, Sept. 26, 1980), p. 64008.

175. Rettig, *Implementing,* p. iii.

176. Harold A. Cohen and Margaret Solnick, "The Financing of CABs," Paper prepared for the *Technology Assessment Forum on Coronary Artery Bypass Surgery: Economic, Ethical and Social Issues* (Washington, D.C.: Sponsored by the National Center for Health Care Technology in collaboration with the National Lung and Blood Institute, April 1981), p. 2.

177. Patricia Roberts Harris, transcript of press conference, June 12, 1980, p. 2.

178. Ibid.

179. *Health Care Financing Review,* Health Care Financing Administration, Department of Health and Human Services, Sept. 182, p. 19, table 1, and HCFA press release, July 18, 1983.

180. *A Profile—Medical Devices and Diagnostic Products Industry* (Washington, D.C.: Pharmaceuticals Manufacturers Association, March 1982), p. 12, table 2, and *Source Book of Health Insurance Data, 1981-82* (Washington, D.C.: Health Insurance Association of America), p. 23, table 2.1, and *PMA 1979-80 Annual Survey Report* (Washington, D.C.: Pharmaceutical Association of America), p. 5, table 1, and ***Prescription Drug Industry*** (Washington, D.C.: Pharmaceuticals Association of America, fact book, 1980), p. 8, table 4, and *Health U.S., 1981,* Health Care Financing Administration, Department of Health and Human Services (pub. no. PHS 82-1232), p. 251, table 53, p. 244, table 47, and press material, security analysts briefing (Milwaukee, Wis.: General Electric Medical Systems, May 5, 1982).

181. Arnold S. Relman, "The New Medical-Industrial Complex," *New England Journal of Medicine,* Oct. 23, 1980, p. 963, and Richard B. Siegrist, Jr., "Wall Street and the For-Profit Hospital Management Companies," *The New Health Care for Profit: Doctors and Hospitals in a Competitive Environment* (Washington, D.C.: Institute of Medicine, National Academy Press, 1983), p. 36.

182. Thomas, *Lives of a Cell,* p. 39.

183. Ibid.

184. *Securing Access to Health Care: The Ethical Implications of Differences in the Availability of Health Services* (Washington, D.C.: President's Commission for the Study of Ethical Problems in Medicine and Biomedical and Behavioral Research, March 1983), vol. 1, p. 84.

BIBLIOGRAPHY

Action for Mental Health: Final Report of the Joint Commission on Mental Illness and Health. New York: Basic Books, 1961.

Alford, Robert R. *Health Care Politics: Ideological and Interest Group Barriers to Reform.* Chicago: University of Chicago Press, 1975.

Altman, Stuart H., and Harvey M. Saposky, eds. *Federal Health Programs: Problems and Prospects.* Lexington, Mass.: Lexington Books, 1981.

Banta, H. David, et al. *Toward Rational Technology in Medicine: Considerations for Health Policy.* New York: Spring Publishing Company, 1981.

Berki, S. F., ed. "Health Policy in America," *The Annals of the American Academy of Political and Social Science.* Beverly Hills: Sage Publications, July 1983.

Brown, Jack H. U. *The Politics of Health Care.* Cambridge, Mass.: Ballinger; Harper & Row, 1978.

Building America's Health: A Report to the President by the President's Commission on the Health Needs of the Nation. Washington, D.C., Dec. 18, 1952.

Califano, Joseph A., Jr. *Governing America: An Insider's Report from the White House and the Cabinet.* New York: Simon and Schuster, 1981.

Carter, Jimmy. *Keeping Faith: Memoirs of a President.* New York: Bantam Books, 1982.

Chu, Franklin D., and Sharland Trotter. *The Madness Establishment: Ralph Nader's Study Group Report on the National Institute of Mental Health.* New York: Grossman, 1974.

Davis, Karen. *National Health Insurance: Benefits, Costs and Consequences.* Washington, D.C.: Brookings Institution, 1975.

Davis, Karen, and Cathy Schoen. *Health and the War on Poverty: A Ten Year Appraisal.* Washington, D.C.: Brookings Institution, 1978.

Derthick, Martha. *Policymaking for Social Security.* Washington, D.C.: Brookings Institution, 1979.

Enthoven, Alain C. *Health Plan: The Only Practical Solution to the Soaring Cost of Medical Care.* Reading, Mass.: Addison-Wesley, 1980.

Falkson, Joseph L. *HMOs and the Politics of Health System Reform.* Chicago: American Hospital Association, 1980.

Feder, Judith, et al., eds. *National Health Insurance: Conflicting Goals and Policy Choices.* Washington, D.C.: Urban Institute Press, 1980.

Fein, Rashi. *The Doctor Shortage: An Economic Diagnosis.* Washington, D.C.: Brookings Institution, 1976.

Foley, Henry A. *Community Mental Health Legislation: The Formative Process.* Lexington, Mass.: Lexington Books, 1975.

Foley, Henry A., and Steven S. Sharfstein. *Madness and Government: Who Cares for the Mentally Ill?* Washington, D.C.: American Psychiatric Press, 1983.

Fox, Rene C., and Judith P. Swazey. *Courage to Fail.* Chicago: University of Chicago Press, 1974, 1978.

Friedman, Kenneth M., and Stuart H. Rakoff, eds. *Toward a National Health Policy: Public Policy and the Control of Health Care Costs.* Lexington, Mass.: Lexington Books, 1977.

Fuchs, Victor R. *Who Shall Live? Health, Economics, and Social Choice.* New York: Basic Books, 1974.

Furman, Bess. *A Profile of the U.S. Public Health Service, 1798-1948.* Washington, D.C.: National Library of Medicine, Department of Health, Education and Welfare. (NIH-73-369)[circa 1973].

Ginzberg, Eli. *The Limits of Health Care Reform: The Search for Realism.* New York: Basic Books, 1977.

Ginzberg, Eli, and Marion Audow. *Men, Money and Medicine.* New York: Columbia University Press, 1965.

Gray, Bradford H., ed. *The New Health Care for Profit: Doctors and Hospitals in a Competitive Environment.* Washington, D.C.: National Academy Press, 1983.

Harris, Richard. *A Sacred Trust.* New York: New American Library, 1966.

Harris, Seymour E. *The Economics of Health Care: Finance and Delivery.* Berkeley, Calif.: McCutchan, 1975.

Havighurst, Clark. *Deregulating the Health Care Industry: Planning for Competition.* Cambridge, Mass.: Ballinger, 1981.

Health Policy: The Legislative Agenda. Washington, D.C.: Congressional Quarterly, 1980.

Heineman, Ben W. Jr., and Curtis A. Hessler. *Memorandum for a President: A Strategic Approach to Domestic Affairs in the 1980s.* New York: Random House, 1980.

Hirshfield, Daniel S. *Lost Reform: The Campaign for Compulsory Health Insurance in the United States from 1932 to 1943.* Cambridge, Mass.: Harvard University Press, 1970.

Holahan, John. *Financing Health Care for the Poor: The Medicaid Experience.* Lexington, Mass.: Lexington Books, 1975.

Kennedy, Edward M. *In Critical Condition: The Crisis in American Health Care.* New York: Simon and Schuster, 1972.

Law, Sylvia. *Blue Cross: What Went Wrong:* New Haven, Conn.: Yale University Press, 1974.

Lindsay, Cotton, ed. *New Directions in Public Health Care: A Prescription for the 1980s.* 3d ed. San Francisco: Institute of Contemporary Studies, 1980.

Magnuson, Warren G. *How Much for Health?* Washington, D.C.: Luce, 1974.

Marmor, Theodore, with Jan Marmor. *Politics of Medicare.* Chicago: Aldine, 1973.

Mechanic, David. *Future Issues in Health Care: Social Policy and the Relations of Medical Services.* New York: Free Press, 1979.

Meyer, Jack. *Health Care Cost Increase.* Washington, D.C.: American Enterprise Institute, 1977.

National Commission on the Cost of Medical Care: 1976-1977. Monroe, Wis.: American Medical Association, 1978.

Neustadt, Richard E., and Harvey V. Fineberg. *Swine Flu Affair: Decision Making on a Slippery Disease.* Washington, D.C.: Department of Health, Education and Welfare, Public Health Service, July 1978.

Newhouse, Joseph P. *The Economics of Medical Care: A Policy Perspective.* Reading, Mass.: Addison-Wesley, 1978.

Olson, Mancor, ed. *A New Approach to the Economics of Health Care.* Washington, D.C.: American Enterprise Institute, 1981.

Palmer, John L., and Isabell V. Sawhill. *The Reagan Experiment.* Washington, D.C.: Urban Institute Press, 1982.

Physicians for a Growing America: Report of the Surgeon General's Consultant Group on Medical Education (Bane Committee). Washington, D.C.: Government Printing Office, 1959.

Redman, Eric. *The Dance of Legislation.* New York: Simon and Schuster, 1973.

Rettig, Richard A. *Implementing the End Stage Renal Disease Program of Medicare.* Prepared for the Health Care Financing Administration, Department of Health, Education and Welfare. (R-2505-HCFA/HEW). Santa Monica, Calif.: Rand Corporation, September 1980.

Russell, Louise B. *Technology in Hospitals: Medical Advances and their Diffusion.* Washington, D.C.: Brookings Institution, 1979.

Schwartz, Harry. *The Case for American Medicine: A Realistic Look at the Health Care System.* New York: McKay, 1972.

Securing Access to Health Care: The Ethical Implications of Differences in the Availability of Health Services. Vol. 1. Report. Washington, D.C.: President's Commission for the Study of Ethical Problems in Medicine and Biomedical and Behavioral Research, March 1983.

Sommers, Anne R. *Rethinking Medicare to Meet Future Needs.* A paper presented to the Government Research Corporation's 7th Annual Leadership Conference on Health Policy, Washington, D.C., June 17, 1982.

Sommers, Anne R., and Herman M. *Health and Health Care: Policies in Perspective.* Rockville, Md.: Aspen Systems Corp., 1977.

Sommers, Herman M., and Anne R. *Medicare and Hospitals: Issues and Prospects.* Washington, D.C.: Brookings Institution, 1967.

Spingarn, Natalie Davis. *Heartbeat: The Politics of Health Research.* Washington, D.C.: Luce, 1976.

Spiegel, Allen D., ed. *Medicaid. Lesson for National Health Insurance.* Rockville, Md.: Aspen Publications, 1975.

Starr, Paul, *The Transformation of American Medicine.* New York: Basic Books, 1982.

Stevens, Rosemary. *American Medicine and the Public Interest.* New Haven, Conn.: Yale University Press, 1971.

Straetz, Ralph A., et. al., eds. *Critical Issues in Health Policy.* Lexington, Mass.: Lexington Books, 1981.

Strickland, Stephen P. *U.S. Health Care: What's Wrong and What's Right.* New York: Universe Books, 1972.

Strickland, Stephen P. *Politics, Science and Dread Disease.* Cambridge, Mass.: Harvard University Press, 1972.

Sundquist, James L. *The Decline and Resurgence of Congress.* Washington, D.C.: Brookings Institution, 1981.

Thomas, Lewis. *The Lives of a Cell: Notes of a Biology Watcher.* New York: Bantam Books, 1974.

Thompson, Frank J. *Health Policy and the Bureaucracy: Politics and Implementation.* Cambridge, Mass.: MIT Press, 1981.

Veatch, Robert A. *Death, Dying and the Biological Revolution: Our Last Quest for Responsibility.* New Haven, Conn.: Yale University Press, 1976.

INDEX

ABOUT THE AUTHOR

Born in Boston in 1933, Jonas Morris lived in nearby Belmont until 1944 when he moved with his parents to Washington, D.C. He attended Hobart College, from which he graduated in 1955, spending the next two years as a deck line officer on a destroyer bouncing about the Pacific Ocean. Following discharge from the Navy in 1957, he worked for newspapers in and about San Francisco, and in 1959 returned to Washington, where for the next several years he worked as a reporter for Congressional Quarterly news service. In 1962 he began a several-year stint at the House of Representatives, working on the professional staff of both congressional committees and members of the House. In 1967 he started a governmental affairs consulting business providing lobbying and other services to public-interest organizations, many of them concerned with federal health programs. During this period he began writing and publishing a newsletter, *Health Systems Report*, on federal health policy. He terminated the lobbying side of his business in 1978 to concentrate on his journalism, and in 1980 he began writing this book. He lives in Washington with his wife, son, and daughter.